Inflammatory Bowel Disease

A Guide for Patients and Their Families

Second Edition

Inflammatory Bowel Disease

A Guide for Patients
and Their Families

—— *Second Edition* ——

Editors

Stanley H. Stein, M.D.
Fort Bend-Brazoria
Gastroenterology Associates
Missouri City, Texas

Richard P. Rood, M.D., F.A.C.P.
Attending Gastroenterologist
Lake Hospital System
Meridia Health System
University Hospitals of Cleveland
Assistant Clinical Professor
  of Medicine
Case Western Reserve University
School of Medicine
Cleveland, Ohio

For the
Crohn's & Colitis Foundation of America, Inc.

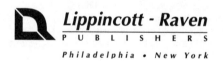

Lippincott - Raven
P U B L I S H E R S
Philadelphia • New York

Acquisitions Editor: Joyce-Rachel John
Developmental Editor: Glenda Insua
Manufacturing Manager: Dennis Teston
Production Manager: Jodi Borgenicht
Production Editor: Catherine Crimi
Cover Designer: Joseph DePinho
Indexer: Lisa Mulleneaux
Compositor: Lippincott–Raven Desktop Division
Printer: RR Donnelley

Printed and bound in the United States of America

9 8 7 6 5 4 3 2 1

Library of Congress Cataloging-in-Publication Data
Inflammatory bowel disease: a guide for patients and their families / edited by Stanley H.
  Stein and Richard P. Rood for the Crohn's & Colitis Foundation of America. —2nd ed.
        p.   cm.
  Includes bibliographical references and index.
  ISBN 0-397-51771-8
    1. Inflammatory bowel disease—Popular works. I. Stein, Stanley H.   II. Rood,
  Richard P. III. Crohn's & Colitis Foundation of America.
RC862.I53I5232   1998
616.3'44—DC21   98-21442
                                                                                     CIP

Care has been taken to confirm the accuracy of the information presented and to describe generally accepted practices. However, the authors, editors, and publisher are not responsible for errors or omissions or for any consequences from application of the information in this book and make no warranty, express or implied, with respect to the contents of the publication.

The authors, editors, and publisher have exerted every effort to ensure that drug selection and dosage set forth in this text are in accordance with current recommendations and practice at the time of publication. However, in view of ongoing research, changes in government regulations, and the constant flow of information relating to drug therapy and drug reactions, the reader is urged to check the package insert for each drug for any change in indications and dosage and for added warnings and precautions. This is particularly important when the recommended agent is a new or infrequently employed drug.

Some drugs and medical devices presented in this publication have Food and Drug Administration (FDA) clearance for limited use in restricted research settings. It is the responsibility of the health care provider to ascertain the FDA status of each drug or device planned for use in their clinical practice.

To all the physician and lay volunteers who spend countless hours of their free time to advance the cause of the CCFA and its mission statement.

To the families of these volunteers, who must also give of their time in the fulfillment of this goal.

S.H.S.

To Shari, Emily, Allison, and David for their support and assistance during the preparation of this manuscript.

R.P.R.

Contents

Contributors

Samuel D. Benjamin, M.D. *Director, University Center for Complementary and Alternative Medicine, Associate Professor of Pediatrics and Family Medicine, State University of New York at Stony Brook Health Sciences Center, Stony Brook, New York 11794-8407*

Benjamin D. Chung, M.D. *Senior Fellow, Department of Gastroenterology, University of Texas–Houston School of Medicine, 6431 Fannin, and University of Texas M.D. Anderson Cancer Center, 1515 Holcombe Boulevard, Houston, Texas 77030*

Tracy L. Hull, M.D. *Staff Surgeon, Department of Colorectal Surgery, Cleveland Clinic Foundation, 9500 Euclid Avenue, Cleveland, Ohio 44195*

Morton L. Katz, Ph.D. *4544 Post Oak Place, #250, Houston, Texas 77027*

Burton I. Korelitz, M.D. *Chief, Department of Gastroenterology, Lenox Hill Hospital, 100 East 77th Street, New York, New York 10021; and Clinical Professor, Department of Medicine, New York University School of Medicine, 550 First Avenue, New York, New York 10016*

Ronald L. Koretz, M.D. *Chief, Division of Gastroenterology, Department of Internal Medicine, Olive View—UCLA Medical Center, 14445 Olive View Drive, Sylmar, California 91342; and Professor, Department of Clinical Medicine, UCLA School of Medicine, 10833 LeConte Avenue, Los Angeles, California 90024*

Bret A. Lashner, M.D. *Director, Department of Gastroenterology, Center for Inflammatory Bowel Disease, Cleveland Clinic Foundation, 9500 Euclid Avenue, Cleveland, Ohio 44195*

Bernard Levin, M.D. *Vice President, Division of Cancer Prevention, and Professor, Department of Gastrointestinal Oncology and Digestive Diseases, University of Texas M.D. Anderson Cancer Center, 1515 Holcombe Boulevard, Box 203, Houston, Texas 77030*

Joel B. Levine, M.D.   *Professor, Department of Medicine, University of Connecticut School of Medicine, 230 Farmington Avenue, Farmington, Connecticut 06030*

Marjorie Merrick   *Director, Department of Research and Education, Crohn's and Colitis Foundation of America, Inc., 386 Park Avenue South, New York, New York 10016-8804*

Guy R. Orangio, M.D., F.A.C.S., F.A.S.C.R.S.   *Chief of Staff, Saint Joseph's Hospital of Atlanta, 5665 Peachtree Dunwoody Road; and Associate Clinical Professor, Medical College of Georgia, 5555 Peachtree Dunwoody Road, Atlanta, Georgia 30342*

Susan N. Peck, R.N., M.S.N.   *Advanced Practice Nurse, Division of Gastroenterology and Nutrition, The Children's Hospital of Philadelphia, 34th and Civic Center Boulevard, Philadelphia, Pennsylvania 19104*

Mark A. Peppercorn, M.D.   *Director, Center for Inflammatory Bowel Disease, Department of Medicine, Beth Israel Deaconess Medical Center, 330 Brookline Avenue, Boston, Massachusetts 02215; and Professor of Medicine, Harvard Medical School, 25 Shattuck Street, Boston, Massachusetts 02115*

David A. Piccoli, M.D.   *Chief, Division of Gastroenterology and Nutrition, The Children's Hospital of Philadelphia, 34th and Civic Center Boulevard; and Associate Professor, Department of Pediatrics, University of Pennsylvania School of Medicine, 36th and Hamilton Walk, Philadelphia, Pennsylvania 19104*

Jane W. Present   *Chairman Emeutus, Crohn's and Colitis Foundation of America, Inc., 386 Park Avenue South, New York, New York 10016-8804*

Lisa H. Richardson   *National Chapter Administration Committee Chairperson, Immediate Past National Education Committee Chairperson, Crohn's and Colitis Foundation of America, Inc., 386 Park Avenue South, New York, New York 10016-8804*

Richard P. Rood, M.D., F.A.C.P.   *Assistant Clinical Professor of Medicine, Case Western Reserve University School of Medicine, Attending Gastroenterologist, Lake Hospital System, Meridia Health System, University Hospitals of Cleveland Center for Digestive Health, Inc., 34940 Ridge Road, Willoughby, Ohio 44094*

Lawrence J. Saubermann, M.D.   *Post-doctoral Research Fellow, Department of Gastroenterology, Brigham and Women's Hospital, 75 Francis Street; and Harvard Medical School, 25 Shattuck Street, Boston, Massachusetts 02115*

Joseph H. Sellin, M.D.   *Chief, Department of Gastroenterology, Memorial Hermann Hospital, 6411 Fannin; Director, Department of Gastroenterology; and Professor, Department of Internal Medicine, University of Texas Houston Health Science Center, 6431 Fannin, Houston, Texas 77030*

Stanley H. Stein, M.D.   *Fort Bend-Brazoria Gastroenterology Associates, 5819 Highway 6 South, #350, Missouri City, Texas 77459*

Jacqueline L. Wolf, M.D.   *Director, Inflammatory Bowel Disease Center, Department of Gastroenterology, Brigham and Women's Hospital, 75 Francis Street; and Associate Professor, Department of Clinical Medicine, Harvard Medical School, 25 Shattuck Street, Boston, Massachusetts 02115*

Foreword

When Dr. Kirsner and I embarked on the first edition of "Inflammatory Bowel Disease: A Guide for Patients and Their Families" we recognized the need for educational material directed towards a lay audience. We believed our effort brought together up-to-date and readable information for the many sufferers of inflammatory bowel disease (IBD). We knew that both those afflicted and their loved ones sought a resource that would explain what was going wrong with their bodies, what they could anticipate for their future health, how the medical profession was diagnosing and treating their conditions, and how others were coping. We attempted to provide a comprehensive and optimistic reference that many have told us they keep by their bedside for insight and comfort.

Unbeknownst to us, at the same time the Crohn's and Colitis Foundation of America (CCFA) (then the National Foundation for Ileitis and Colitis [NFIC]) was preparing a somewhat similar reference, "The Crohn's and Colitis Fact Book." In a more topic-related, question-and-answer format, the "Fact Book" became a complementary companion to our "Guide."

The time has come to update both books. As the CCFA has grown, and the medical and scientific community has become even more involved via the Patient Education Committee of the National Scientific Cabinet, we were delighted to hand over the task of updating and combining the two books. Under the direction of Dr. Stanley Stein, the Patient Education Committee has taken on the challenge and solicited a marvelous group of physicians, nurses, dieticians, CCFA leaders and patients to create a modern reference that should serve the public for the next decade.

Of course, what is critically needed is the collaborative clinical and basic research to identify the causes and cures for these chronic intestinal disorders that afflict men and women of all ages and ethnicities, but particularly the young. We fully anticipate that in the next decade we will elucidate the genetic underpinnings and environmental triggers that culminate in IBD. We are hopeful that the next edition will place the causes in a historical context and focus on the cures.

Stephen B. Hanauer, M.D.
Co-Director, IBD Research Center
Professor, Department of Medicine and
Clinical Pharmacology
University of Chicago
Chicago, Illinois

Preface

This book developed as an extension of the recent updating of the Crohn's and Colitis Foundation of America (CCFA) pamphlets for newly diagnosed patients. Although the previous Fact Book was extremely informative and helpful to a countless number of patients, through time it became apparent that it urgently needed updating. As Dr. Steven Hanauer was gracious enough to give the Foundation the right to his patient book, we used this as a base from which to build and expand upon for a second edition.

The efforts put into these pages were those of a labor of love for all involved. This book is intended to be user-friendly for the patient; that is, unlike medical textbooks where you may have to look at three or four different chapters to find one subject, each chapter in this guide is self-sufficient and can stand on its own. This format was intended to facilitate quick and easy reference. In response to numerous questions from patients, we have also added a chapter on alternative medicine to make this guide a more complete resource.

We gratefully acknowledge the authors and members of the committee that developed this work, and thank them for their thoroughness and attentiveness to detail.

Inflammatory Bowel Disease

A Guide for Patients and Their Families

Second Edition

CHAPTER 1

ANATOMY AND FUNCTION

Joseph H. Sellin and *Benjamin D. Chung

THE DIGESTIVE SYSTEM

The digestive system refers to all of the organs involved with the digestion, absorption, and metabolism of nutrients. The digestive tract is a continuous tube beginning from the mouth, coursing through the body, ultimately ending at the anus. The digestive system can be divided into several anatomic regions as shown in Table 1 (Fig. 1). The main functions of the digestive system are (a) absorption of nutrients, (b) maintenance of fluid balance, (c) excretion of waste, and (d) forming a barrier as protection from a hostile environment.

---

*Department of Internal Medicine, University of Texas Houston Health Science Center, Department of Gastroenterology, Memorial Hermann Hospital, Houston, Texas 77030; and *Department of Gastroenterology, University of Texas M.D. Anderson Cancer Center, and University of Texas—Houston School of Medicine, Houston, Texas 77030*

TABLE 1. *The digestive system*

I. The digestive tract
  Oral cavity
  Oral pharynx
  Esophagus
  Stomach
  Small intestine
    Duodenum
    Jejunum
    Ileum
  Large intestine
    Ascending colon
    Transverse colon
    Descending colon
    Sigmoid
    Rectum
    Anus
II. Other specialized organs
  Salivary glands
  Liver
  Gallbladder
  Pancreas

The Oral Cavity and Oropharynx

The oral cavity consists of the lips, teeth, gums, tongue, cheeks, palate (roof of the mouth), floor of the mouth, and salivary glands. As a whole, the oral cavity performs chewing (called *mastication*) by means of an intricate coordination of its components. Mastication crushes food particles into smaller, more manageable forms. During this process, the initial digestion of some nutrients begins in the oral cavity. Mastication also stimulates the taste buds of the tongue and releases the odor of the food particles, thereby stimulating the olfactory (smell) nerves of the brain. This plays an important role in the pleasure of eating. The muscles involved in mastication are some of the most powerful in the body, producing pressures up to 60 to 200 pounds on the molars. The oropharynx refers to the throat. The various muscles of the oropharynx coordinate the swallowing reflex, a process called *deglutition*. The main function of the oropharynx is to transfer food from the oral cavity to the esophagus.

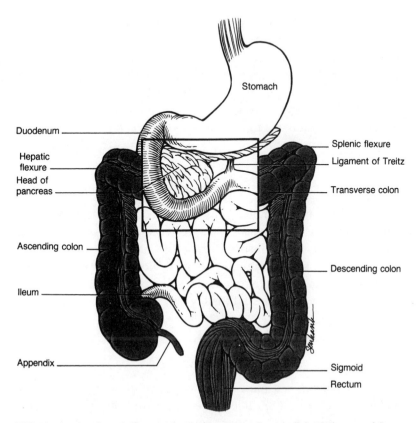

FIG. 1. Anatomic relations among the stomach, small intestine, and large intestine. (From Rubin D. Small intestine: anatomy and structural anomalies. In: Yamada T, Owyang C, Powell DW, Silverstein FE, eds. *Textbook of gastroenterology,* 2nd ed. Philadelphia: Lippincott-Raven Publishers, 1995;1556.)

Saliva

Three glands in the oral cavity (parotid, sublingual, and submandibular) secrete between 1 and 1.5 L (approximately 0.3 to 0.4 gallons) of saliva each day. Most saliva is swallowed and handled by the rest of the digestive tract. Saliva contains *salivary amylase*, an enzyme that begins the digestion of ingested carbohydrates within the oral cavity, and *mucin*, which accounts for the mucous characteristic of saliva. Mucin's main role is to provide lubrication of the food particles before swallowing. Salivary secretion can be stimulated by either the food particles in the oral cavity or the impulses from the higher centers of the brain such as a thought of food. Also contained in the saliva are other enzymes called lysozymes and certain antibodies to help fight off potential infections. Swallowed saliva is alkaline and helps neutralize the acid that may reflux (flow back) from the stomach to the esophagus, protecting it from damage by gastric (stomach) acid.

Enzyme

An enzyme is a complex protein produced by the body's cells and is involved in numerous chemical reactions necessary for the body's normal metabolism. During the chemical reactions, an enzyme can change, combine, or break down various molecules such as nutrients. An example is the salivary amylase (see above), which breaks down (digests) the ingested carbohydrates in the oral cavity.

Esophagus

The esophagus is a muscular tube that connects the oropharynx and the stomach. Its typical length is approximately 25 cm (about 10 in.), whereas its diameter ranges between 1.5 and 2 cm. The body of the esophagus is made up of two layers of muscle; the inner muscles are circular, whereas the outer muscles run along the length of the esophagus. The coordinated contractions of the esophageal muscles during the swallowing process, called *peristalsis*, propels food into the stomach and subsequently through the intestine.

The esophagus also has two regions called *sphincters*, which play an important role in moving the ingested food in the correct direction, i.e., toward the stomach. They are formed by certain circular muscles around and within the body of the esophagus. The upper esophageal sphincter is located just below the oropharynx, whereas the lower sphincter is located in the lower portion of the esophagus just above the stomach. Impaired function of the lower esophageal sphincter can allow backflow (*reflux*) of the stomach's acid, contributing to heartburn. *Belching* is a process of expulsion of swallowed air from the stomach that results when the lower esophageal sphincter relaxes to allow backflow of the stomach contents. The esophagus is normally empty except during a meal.

Stomach

The stomach serves as both a reservoir and a blender of ingested food. It consists of three main parts: fundus, body, and the antrum (Fig. 2). The upper portion of the stomach, the *fundus* and the *body*, mainly serves as a reservoir. The stomach can expand its volume from about 50 mL during fasting to as large as 2 L after a meal in a process called *receptive relaxation*. The *antrum* is the funnel-shaped lower portion of the stomach. Its forceful contractions grind the ingested food and mix it with the stomach's secretions such as acid and digestive enzymes. Only after the food particles are crushed into an acceptable size do they pass into the small intestine through the *pylorus*, a valve at the lowermost part of the stomach. Although the stomach grinds, digests, and empties the final product, *chyme*, into

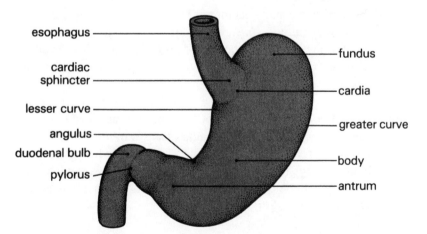

FIG. 2. Diagram of the stomach and its three main anatomic parts: fundus, body, and antrum. The upper and lower curvatures of the stomach are called lesser and greater curvatures, respectively. (From Eastwood G.L. Stomach: anatomy and structural anomalies. In: Yamada T, Owyang C, Powell DW, Silverstein FE, eds. *Textbook of gastroenterology*, 2nd ed. Philadelphia: Lippincott-Raven Publishers, 1995;1304.)

the small intestine, very little absorption of nutrients occurs in the stomach.

The stomach is a remarkable organ. It is able to handle the various forms of food or even an ingested foreign body at different times while maintaining its primary role in digestion. During fasting, the stomach is relatively quiet; once a person begins to perceive hunger, however, certain forms of contractions begin to appear in preparation for a new meal ("hunger pangs").

The stomach produces up to 2 to 2.5 L of secretions each day. The secretions contain various products such as *acid* and *pepsin,* both of which are involved in the digestion of proteins. In addition, the stomach secretes *gastrin*, a hormone that stimulates acid secretion, and *intrinsic factor*, a cofactor responsible for the absorption of vitamin B_{12}.

The stomach normally has several lines of defense against various insults from the outside world. From an evolutionary perspective, gastric acid is one of the first lines of protection against potentially dangerous infectious agents. At the same time, however, the stomach must protect itself from being digested by the acid that it secretes. Against all these, the stomach maintains a protective layer of mucus and alkaline bicarbonate on its lining. The stomach also secretes substances called *prostaglandins*, which are thought to stimulate the secretion of mucus and bicarbonate and promote blood flow. In addition, the lining cells of the stomach constantly repair any injuries that they sustain.

Nevertheless, a breakdown of the stomach's defense mechanisms can occur in the face of the numerous insults and may lead to *peptic ulcer disease*, one of the most common diseases in the world. Other examples of external assaults damaging to the gastric lining are anti-inflammatory drugs (such as aspirin and ibuprofen), steroids (such as prednisone), alcohol, smoking, and infection by a bacterium called *Helicobacter pylori*.

Small Intestine

The small intestine consists of three parts: duodenum, jejunum, and ileum. With average length somewhere between 22 and 25 feet, it is the longest part of the digestive tract. It begins with the duodenum and ends at the ileocecal valve, through which the intestinal contents enter the large intestine. The average diameter of the small intestine is about 3 to 4 cm (1.5 to 1.8 in.). The inner surface of the small intestine has numerous small folds and ridges on its lining called *valvulae conniventes*. These folds increase the surface area by about fivefold.

A cross-section of the small intestine (Fig. 3) is divided into four layers: serosa, muscularis, submucosa, and mucosa. The *serosa*, the

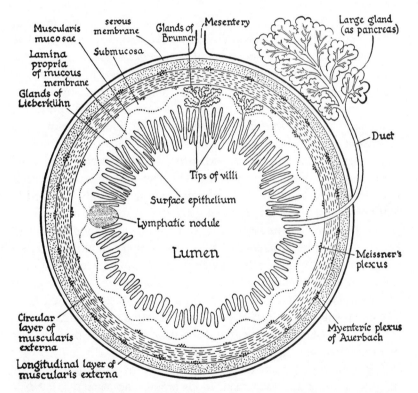

FIG. 3. A cross-section of the small intestine. The outermost layer (serosa) is a thin membrane that surrounds the inner layer (muscularis) containing numerous networks of nerve fibers called plexus. Various glands are found in the submucosa and the mucosa. Pancreatic juices drain into the intestinal lumen through a specialized tube (pancreatic duct). (From Trier JS, Winter HS. Small intestinal anatomy and development abnormalities. In: Sleisenger MH, Fordtran JS, eds. *Gastrointestinal disease.* Philadelphia: WB Saunders, 1993;794.)

outermost layer, is an extension of the membrane that lines the abdominal cavity called *peritoneum*. The next layer is the *muscularis*, which consists of two layers of muscle. The outer layer muscle runs along the length of the intestine, whereas the inner layer is circular along the circumference of the intestine. This arrangement is similar to that of the esophagus. The countless nerve fibers in this region control the movements of the muscles and propel the nutrients and other contents downstream. The next layer is called *submucosa* and contains connective tissues, various immune cells, and blood vessels.

The innermost layer is the *mucosa*, which makes up the lining of the intestine. The mucosa is divided into even smaller sublayers. The outermost sublayer of mucosa is called *muscularis mucosa* (separate from the muscularis above), consisting of a thin sheet of muscle. The next sublayer is called *lamina propria*. This is an important sublayer containing numerous immune cells responsible for intestinal immune responses to foreign substances. In addition, numerous microscopic blood vessels (capillaries) and lymph vessels exist here and transport the nutrients absorbed by the villous epithelial cells (see below) to other parts of the body. The innermost sublayer is lined by the *epithelial cells*. This layer contains the cells involved in nutrient absorption and the goblet cells, which secrete mucus.

The lining of the intestine is covered with tiny (about 1 mm in height) finger-like projections called *villi*, which contain the epithelial cells. The surface of these projections are, in turn, covered with even smaller, microscopic projections known as *microvilli* (Fig. 4). These structures increase the surface area even further by 500-fold. The end result is an enormous inner surface area of about 250 m^3. It is through this huge surface area that the small intestine performs its main function, i.e., absorption of nutrients.

The *duodenum* is the first part of the small intestine about 9 to 11 in. long forming a C shape as it loops around the pancreas. Pancreatic juice and bile drain into the duodenum through an opening called the ampulla of Vater. The *jejunum* immediately follows the duodenum. With its average length of 8 feet, it makes up two fifths of the length of the small intestine. The next part is the *ileum*. There is no discrete point where jejunum ends and ileum begins. The ileum is narrower, and its wall is thinner than the jejunum. The last part of

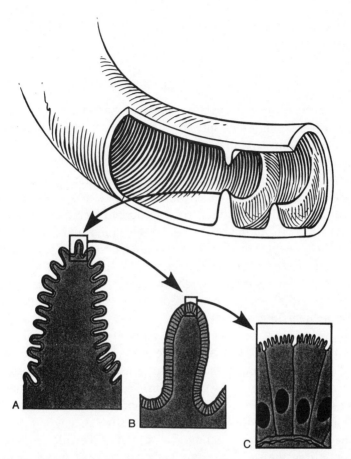

FIG. 4. The lining of the small intestine. The folds of the lining of the small intestine (valvulae conniventes) **(A)**, increase the inner surface area by five-fold. These folds contain finger-like villi **(B)**, which, in turn, contain numerous microvilli **(C)**, increasing the total inner surface area of the small intestine by 500-fold. (From Bloom WN, Fawcett DW. *A textbook of histology*. New York: Chapman and Hall, 1968.)

the ileum (*terminal ileum*) is where the absorption of vitamin B_{12} and most of the secreted bile acids occurs. Although *Crohn's disease* (CD) can involve any part of the digestive tract, this is the most commonly involved site. The *ileocecal valve* is the point where the small intestine ends and the large intestine begins. As its name suggests, it serves to prevent backflow (reflux) of contents from the large intestine to the ileum.

Large Intestine

The large intestine, also called the colon, has an average length of 4 to 5 feet. Like the small intestine, there are several sections of the colon, which are structurally similar but have somewhat different functions. These consist of the cecum, ascending colon, transverse colon, sigmoid, rectum, and anus (Fig. 1). The colon's primary functions are to absorb water and electrolytes and to propel its contents, including byproducts of digestion, unabsorbed fibers, and mucus, to their final exit from the body. Unlike the stomach and small intestine, which are relatively sterile, the colon harbors a large population of bacteria that normally reside (known as the *normal flora)* in the lumen (the hollow space inside the intestine). Human feces contains about 10 billion organisms per gram of stool. This represents approximately 25% of fecal weight!

The colon also has outer muscles along its length and inner, circular muscles. A cross-section of the colon is similar to that of the small intestine and consists of serosa, muscularis, submucosa, and mucosa. The innermost layer, *mucosa*, contains cells that absorb water and electrolytes as well as mucus-producing cells. The colon does not have villi nor does it contain digestive enzymes.

The *cecum* is the first and the widest part of the colon, where the contents from the small intestine drain through the ileocecal valve. The *appendix* is also attached to the cecum. Although its average length is about 8 cm, the appendix can be as long as 20 cm. The appendix is rich with immune cells. Despite our understanding of its anatomy, the function of the appendix remains largely unknown. When its lumen becomes obstructed (with, for example, fecal materials), inflammation and infection may ensue and *appendicitis* develops.

The *ascending colon*, which follows the cecum, is approximately 8 in. long and arbitrarily ends at the bend of the colon near the liver called the *hepatic flexure.* The next part is the *transverse colon*, which begins from the hepatic flexure and ends at the area near the spleen called the *splenic flexure.* This part is mobile and can drop into the lower abdomen when standing up.

The *descending colon* begins at the splenic flexure and continues downward on the left side of the abdominal cavity until it meets with the *sigmoid colon.* The sigmoid makes a couple of sharp bends as it descends into the pelvis and meets the *rectum.* The rectum is approximately 5 in. long. It plays an important role in the control of defecation. The *anus* is the terminal portion of the large intestine. It is about 1.5 in. long and contains sphincter muscles that control the passage of fecal materials.

OTHER SPECIALIZED ORGANS

Pancreas

The pancreas is in the midline of the abdomen behind and below the stomach and has an average length between 5 and 6 in. (Fig. 5).

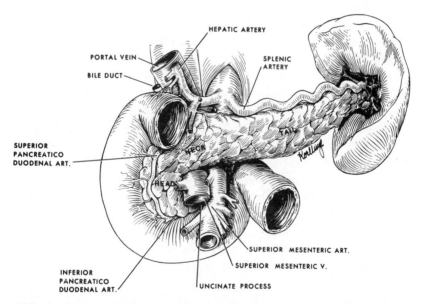

FIG. 5. The pancreas is an elongated structure about 5 to 6 inches in length. Its head and neck are surrounded by the duodenum, which makes a C-shaped loop, and several major blood vessels. The tail of the pancreas ends at the spleen. The bile ducts and the pancreatic ducts course through the pancreas. (From Ermak TH, Grendel JH. The pancreas: anatomy, histology, embryology, and developmental anomalies. In: Sleisenger MH, Fordtran JS, eds. *Gastrointestinal disease.* Philadelphia: WB Saunders, 1993;1574.)

Because it secretes a wide variety of substances, the pancreas can regulate many metabolic processes. There are two general mechanisms of secretion: exocrine and endocrine. When pancreatic cells release their products directly into a system of ducts within the pancreas, this is termed *exocrine* secretion. The system of ducts are like tributaries to a river; they eventually drain through the ampulla of Vater into the small intestine.

The exocrine secretions, the pancreatic juices, measure about 1200 to 1500 mL/day. The key ingredients of pancreatic juices include water, electrolytes, bicarbonate, and enzymes involved in digestion of carbohydrates (pancreatic amylases), protein (trypsin, chymotrypsin), and fat (pancreatic lipase). These are released in response to food in the mouth, stomach, small intestine, or even a thought or smell of food. Hormones and nerves that innervate the pancreas are essential for the regulation of the release of the pancreatic juices.

The second function of the pancreas is called *endocrine* because the secretion products (*hormones*) are directly released into the rich supply of tiny blood vessels in the pancreatic tissue and circulate to distant sites in the body, where they regulate important metabolic functions. The endocrine products are produced by numerous islets of cells found in the pancreas. These islet cells produce *insulin* and *glucagon*. These are hormones that play vital roles in the metabolism of carbohydrates; glucagon stimulates the release of glucose and fatty acids into the bloodstream, whereas insulin stimulates the uptake of glucose into various organs such as the liver and the muscle. Failure to produce adequate amount of insulin accounts for certain forms of *diabetes*.

The pancreas can become inflamed, a condition called pancreatitis. Alcohol and gallstones are the most common causes of pancreatitis. The condition can be acute and self-limited or chronic.

Liver

The liver is the largest organ in the body, weighing somewhere between 1200 and 1500 g and is about 2.5% of the total body weight. It is found in the upper right part of the abdomen. In its vicinity run the right kidney, colon (hepatic flexure of the colon), duodenum, and stomach (Fig. 1). The liver is largely divided into *right* and *left lobes*, with the right lobe being about 6 times bigger than the left lobe. The liver is a highly vascular organ with two blood supplies, i.e., the portal vein and the hepatic artery.

The liver has numerous functions including metabolism of carbohydrates, fat, and proteins; production of numerous proteins, including albumin and blood clotting factors, removal of old, worn-out red blood cells; and detoxification and modification of ingested drugs or any harmful substances. Alcohol is metabolized by the liver. Its chronic use can ultimately lead to scarring (cirrhosis) and liver failure. Various types of viruses can also infect the liver and can cause chronic inflammation and, ultimately, failure. Among these viruses are *hepatitis A, B* and *C*, three of the most common diseases in the world.

The liver also makes *bile* secreted through the *bile ducts* and stored in the gallbladder, which ultimately drain into the duodenum through the ampulla of Vater. Obstruction of bile flow due to tumors in the liver or pancreas and gallstones in the bile ducts can lead to jaundice. In addition, there are conditions in which the bile ducts become chronically inflamed such as *primary sclerosing cholangitis* (PSC). Curiously, a large percentage of PSC patients are found to have inflammatory bowel disease (IBD). The incidence of ulcerative colitis and CD in patients with PSC is about 70% and 7%, respectively. On the other hand, however, only about 5% of patients with ulcerative colitis and 1% of patients with CD have PSC.

Gallbladder

The gallbladder is a pear-shaped organ located just below the right lobe of the liver. Its main function is to serve as a reservoir of bile until hormonal and neural signals initiated by eating and digestion stimulate the gallbladder to contract and empty its contents into the bile ducts. About 50 mL of bile is normally stored in the gallbladder. Precipitation of bile contents such as cholesterol can result in gallstones.

ABSORPTION OF NUTRIENTS

The three main types of nutrients that supply energy for the body are carbohydrates, fat, and protein (Table 2). In the body, the absorp-

TABLE 2. *Three main types of nutrients*

	Daily contribution to total calories (%)	Daily intake (g)
Carbohydrate	40–45	250–800
Fat	40–45	100–150
Protein	10–15	50–70

tion of nutrients depends on (a) peristalsis to keep things moving downstream, (b) digestion in the intestinal lumen, and (c) absorption of the nutrients through the intestinal wall. *Maldigestion* occurs if any part of the normal digestive process in the lumen is impaired. For example, patients with chronic pancreatitis cannot produce adequate amount of pancreatic enzymes to digest the nutrients and develop maldigestion. Impaired bile secretion (from obstruction, for example) can result in fat maldigestion.

Similarly, *malabsorption* occurs when any part of the absorption process through the intestinal wall (lining) is defective. An example is *lactase deficiency*, which is one of the most common causes of malabsorption in the world affecting particularly Asians, native and black Americans, and about 20% of white Americans. Lactase is an enzyme found on the intestinal lining cells (see section under carbohydrates) that breaks down lactose, a common sugar found in milk. Thus, persons with *lactase deficiency* have lactose malabsorption and develop common symptoms of abdominal cramps, bloating, and diarrhea. A variety of diseases affecting the small bowel can also lead to an acquired form of lactase deficiency, including CD.

Carbohydrates

The most common forms of carbohydrates obtained in the human diet are starch (about 50%), lactose, and sucrose. *Starch* comes from plants and is made up of long chains of glucose. *Lactose* (made of two simple sugars bound to each other: glucose and galactose) is found in milk. *Sucrose* (made of glucose and fructose) is found in sugar cane.

The digestion of carbohydrates begins in the mouth. The salivary glands release enzymes called *salivary amylases* into the mouth during mastication (enzymes are complex proteins that serve as cata-lysts in various chemical reactions in the body). These enzymes break down the carbohydrates into smaller fragments of varying sizes, which can range from *disaccharides* (made up of two sugar molecules) to somewhat larger molecules called *oligosaccharides* (each containing several sugar molecules). After the partially digested carbohydrates as well as food particles with intact carbohy-drates enter the stomach, amylase become inactivated by gastric acid. Once in the stomach, the food particles are ground and blended with stomach secretions. The resulting partially digested food in the stomach, called *chyme*, enters the duodenum, where further diges-tion of remaining carbohydrates continues.

The processing of chyme in the small intestine consists of two parts. First, the nutrients including carbohydrates are digested by the enzymes in the pancreatic juice (*pancreatic amylase* breaks down complex carbohydrates into simple sugars). Second, the nutrients are further digested and then absorbed by the lining cells of the intestine.

Carbohydrates must be completely broken down to single sugar molecules (e.g., glucose) for absorption to occur. Therefore, the end products of the pancreatic amylase action in the lumen, disaccha-rides and oligosaccharides, are further digested by other enzymes found on the villi of the small intestine, particularly the duodenum and the jejunum. These enzymes are called *brush border enzymes* (brush border refers to the inner lining layer containing the villi). Their actions release single sugar molecules.

The three main single sugar molecules released this way are *glu-cose, galactose* (from milk), and *fructose* (from sugar canes and fruits). These single sugar molecules are then absorbed by specific transport mechanisms. Once they are absorbed, they are then released into the bloodstream to circulate throughout the body to be taken up by different cells for their metabolism.

Fat

Approximately 90% of an average person's dietary fat is in the form of *triglycerides*. The remaining 10% includes *cholesterol* and *phospholipids*. The main steps of fat digestion are (a) breaking fat into tiny droplets (*emulsification*), (b) dissolving the digested products into *micelles,* (c) digestion of emulsified fat by pancreatic enzymes in the lumen (*lipolysis*), and (d) absorption by the intestinal lining cells.

The main challenge of digestion of fat is that fat does not mix with water. This characteristic of fat is easily visualized by remembering the fat droplets on chicken soup. To deal with this problem, the gut has created a system to dissolve fat in the water of intestinal juices.

Most of the digestion of fat occurs in the small intestine. By the time dietary fat leaves the stomach, it has been *emulsified* into tiny fat droplets. These fat droplets require *bile acids* from the liver and dietary *phospholipids* on their surface to keep them stable, whereas pancreatic lipase acts on the surface of these droplets. The digestive action on the surface of these fat droplets by *pancreatic lipase* breaks the triglycerides down into simpler fats (*fatty acids* and *monoglycerides*). The digestion of these fat droplets by the enzymes is known as *lipolysis.*

As lipolysis proceeds, the fat droplets become progressively smaller as they release the digested products, *fatty acids, monoglycerides*, and *cholesterol* into the lumen. In order for these products to travel across all of the water in the lumen to reach the lining cells for absorption, bile acids from the liver dissolve them by surrounding these molecules, forming even smaller (up to 5 to 10 times smaller than the emulsified fat droplets), microscopic droplets called *mixed micelles,* which are composed of bile acids on the outside with an interior that contains fatty acids, monoglycerides, and cholesterol. Once formed, the mixed micelles deliver their contents into close proximity of the inner lining cells membrane. The fatty acids, monoglycerides, and cholesterol are then released here and absorbed by the lining cells of the intestine.

Bile

Bile is produced by the liver cells and the cells of the bile duct and consists of water, electrolytes, bile acids, bilirubin, cholesterol, and phospholipids. About 500 mL is secreted each day. Some bile is stored in the gallbladder during fasting and released after a meal. Bile acids are essential for the absorption of fat as well as fat-soluble vitamins. After being released into the duodenum through the ampulla of Vater, bile acids travel downstream until they reach the terminal ileum, where most of them (about 90%) are reabsorbed. They then return to the liver via the bloodstream. The bile acids circulate throughout the body this way 6 to 8 times a day. Small amounts of bile are lost in the feces and thus impart the yellowish color of the feces.

Protein

The average daily intake of protein in the United States is about 70 g/day. Dietary proteins, however, only make up 50% to 75% of total proteins absorbed by the small intestine. The rest comes from endogenous sources such as saliva, pancreatic juices, and shedding of the inner lining cells of the intestine. During digestive process, proteins are broken down to smaller units called *dipeptides* (made of two amino acids), *tripeptides* (three amino acids), and so on. *Amino acids* are the basic building blocks of proteins. Bound together by chemical bonds, they form peptides, which, in turn, form various proteins necessary for the body's metabolism.

The digestion of protein consists of two main steps: (a) digestion in the lumen of the stomach and the small intestine by pancreatic enzymes; and (b) further digestion and absorption by the lining cells. The stomach's digestive enzyme, *pepsin*, accounts for about 10% of total protein digestion. The remainder is handled by the pancreatic enzymes (*trypsin, chymotrypsin, elastase,* and *exopeptidases*).

The final products (amino acids, dipeptides, and peptides of several amino acids) of the digestive actions of the enzymes in the lumen then reach the small intestine's lining. Here, the brush border enzymes further digest some of the peptides and release single amino acids and smaller peptides. These are then absorbed by the inner lining cells of the small intestine by specific transport mechanisms. About 10% of the absorbed proteins are used by these cells themselves, whereas the rest are exported elsewhere throughout the body.

Vitamins

Vitamins are complex molecules that are essential in many metabolic processes in the body. They are divided into water-soluble and fat-soluble because they differ in their absorption by the body. The water-soluble vitamins include vitamin C, folic acid, thiamine, riboflavin, pantothenic acid, biotin, pyridoxine, niacin, and vitamin B_{12}. Except for vitamin B_{12}, most of the water-soluble vitamins are absorbed in the proximal small intestine, especially the jejunum. Vitamin B_{12} absorption follows a more complex mechanism in the terminal ileum. The fat-soluble vitamins include vitamins A, D, E, and K. Their absorption parallels that of fat involving the bile acids. Some examples are as follows:

Vitamin C is found in fresh fruits and fruit juices and is absorbed by an active transport by the absorptive cells in the small intestine. Its deficiency causes scurvy. *Thiamine* (vitamin B_1) is found in cereals, beans, and nuts. It is absorbed by the intestinal lining cells. Its deficiency causes impaired neurologic functions. *Riboflavin* (vitamin B_2) is found in liver, milk, and green vegetables. It is involved in the synthesis of certain enzymes and in normal growth. *Pyridoxine* (vitamin B_6) is involved in certain amino acid metabolism. It is absorbed by simple diffusion into the lining cells.

Sources of *folic acid* include spinach, peanuts, and beans. Its dietary source requires action by certain brush border enzymes (hydrolases) and the product is absorbed by the lining cells. The hydrolysis by the enzymes and the absorption are inhibited by *sulfasalazine,* an important and commonly prescribed drug used to treat IBD. Chronic alcohol use also impairs the enzyme activity. Folic acid supplements are often necessary in these situations. Folic acid deficiency causes anemia.

Vitamin B_{12}, also known as cobalamin, is also a water-soluble vitamin. Unlike the others, its absorption is more complex. In the duodenum, dietary vitamin B_{12} binds to a specific protein, *intrinsic factor*, secreted by the stomach. Together they travel downstream to the terminal ileum, where the vitamin is released and absorbed by the lining cells.

The *fat-soluble vitamins* include vitamins A, D, E, and K. They are absorbed in a similar manner as that of fat and occurs in the proximal small intestine. *Vitamin A* is found in milk products and leafy vegetables. It is involved in maintaining cell membranes and night vision. *Vitamin D* is found in certain fish oil (such as tuna and salmon) and is also synthesized by the body with the help of sun exposure. *Vitamin E* is found in vegetables, eggs, and margarine. *Vitamin K* is found in green vegetables. Its deficiency causes impaired functioning of clotting factors and leads to bleeding disorder.

Minerals

Dairy products are important sources of *calcium*. Calcium is absorbed throughout the gut, but most efficiently in the duodenum. Vitamin D stimulates calcium absorption, whereas certain medications such as steroids inhibit intestinal calcium absorption. Chronic use of steroids can, therefore, result in osteoporosis and bone fractures.

Dietary sources of *iron* are meat products and grains. Iron absorption occurs mostly in the proximal small intestine. Iron is an essential part of hemoglobin, found in the red blood cells, which carries oxygen throughout the body. Blood loss from the digestive tract is an important cause of iron deficiency anemia.

FLUID BALANCE

An average person's daily fluid input into the digestive tract is approximately 9 L. It is surprising that the majority of this fluid is not from diet but from the secretions of the intestinal tract itself. The secretions from within the digestive tract constitutes about 7 L, whereas oral intake is only about 1.5 to 2 L (Table 3).The intestinal tract is highly efficient in reabsorbing water and electrolytes. The

TABLE 3. *Daily fluid balance of the digestive tract*

Source	Average intake (mL)	Secreted (mL)	Absorbed (mL)
Dietary	1500–2000		
Saliva		1500	
Gastric secretion		2500	
Pancreatic secretion		1500	
Biliary		500	
Small intestine		1000	7000
Large intestine			>>1500
Total	1500–2000	7000	>8500

lining cells of the small intestine are designed to absorb salt, sugars, and amino acids efficiently, pulling water across the relatively leaky lining cells. Further downstream in the digestive tract the lining becomes tighter. In the colon most of the remaining fluids are absorbed (approximately 1500 mL) with a net excretion of only 100 to 150 mL of fluid in the feces. An important feature of the large intestine is that it has a large capacity to increase its absorption of fluid upon demand (Table 3). Any extra fluid intake in the diet is easily handled by the colon by increasing its absorption, and thus the net output remains relatively unchanged. Certain diseases such as IBD, viral infections, bacterial infections such as cholera, or medications, however, can overwhelm the system and result in diarrhea.

EXCRETION OF WASTE

Defecation

Defecation is the means of ridding the body of intestinal waste. It is controlled by both voluntary and involuntary reflexes. When fecal material reaches the rectum, the sensation activates nerves, which relax the *inner sphincter muscle* in the anus, while tightening the *external sphincter muscle*. A signal is then sent to the brain to generate the urge to defecate. One can voluntarily relax the external sphincter muscle to expel the feces (defecation) or constrict it to hold the feces until a later time.

Intestinal Gas

The main sources of intestinal gas include swallowed air and gas generated by bacterial breakdown of undigested nutrients in the colon. Up to 7 to 10 L of gas is produced each day. Most of the gas in the stomach is swallowed air and is expelled by *belching*. Intestinal gas further downstream is eliminated as *flatus*. The vast majority (about 99%) of flatus consists of odorless nitrogen (swallowed), carbon dioxide (ingested in diet or byproduct of metabolism), oxygen (swallowed), hydrogen (byproduct of bacterial action), and methane (byproduct of bacterial action). It is the trace amount of other gases (ammonia, hydrogen sulfide, etc.) produced by bacterial action on undigested nutrients that accounts for the odor of colonic gas.

BARRIER FUNCTION

An important but less well recognized function of the digestive tract is to provide a barrier function against intruding pathogenic organisms such as bacteria and viruses. This function must entail a fine balance between two opposing forces. On one hand, the intestine must recognize and neutralize the pathogenic organisms. The opposite aspect is the business of recognizing numerous foreign antigens included in ingested food particles that are harmless to the body and develop a tolerance to these foreign bodies. This might explain why the normal intestinal tract harbors a continuous low level of inflammation.

The digestive tract has multiple sites and levels of built-in defense lines against potential pathogens. For example, the saliva contains certain enzymes (lysozymes) and antibodies (IgA) that neutralize pathogens. In addition, the acid and the proteolytic enzymes in the stomach as discussed above are powerful antipathogen mechanisms. The lining cells of the intestines and the mucous layer above them also serve as barriers. The saliva and intestinal secretions, water, and electrolytes also help flush the organisms downstream and eventually excreted. Obviously, the normal contractile movements *(peristalsis)* also assist in propelling the harmful organisms downstream. As previously discussed, the intestine, mostly the large intestine, harbors a large population of organisms that normally reside in the lumen (the "normal flora"). These organisms also play an important role in preventing pathogenic organisms from taking root.

The lamina propria (see above) of the intestinal wall contains various immune cells such as lymphocytes, macrophages, plasma cells, eosinophils, mast cells, and neutrophils. In addition, various chemicals known as *cytokines* are released by the lymphocytes and monocytes. These chemicals stimulate the production of even more lymphocytes. They also can induce the growth of certain cells involved in tissue repair. All of these processes act in concert to fight the infecting organisms. Recent studies have shown that the nervous system in the intestinal tract is also intricately involved in the regulation of immune responses.

A derangement of any of the above processes can lead to problems. For example, failure to develop adequate levels of immunoglobulin A (IgA) can result in bacterial infection. Failure of eosinophil and mast cell response in the intestinal tract can make one susceptible to parasite infections. Inadequate levels of certain lymphocytes (CD4) can lead to numerous opportunistic infections of the gut as seen in autoimmune deficiency syndrome (AIDS).

Loss of the fine regulation and balance of the immune processes can lead to other problems. Antibodies against the body's own cells can result in certain forms of gastritis, an inflammation of the lining of the stomach. The body's cellular immune responses involving lymphocytes, macrophages, and neutrophils against an as yet unknown antigen is thought to be the basis of IBD.

CONCLUSION

Contrary to the simple concept of a continuous tube from the mouth coursing through the body ending at the anus, the digestive system is a complex integration of the body's nervous, immune, endocrine, and circulatory systems. Its metabolic functions and regulations are intricately intertwined at local as well as systemic levels affecting the entire body. Injury or impaired functioning of its various parts cause some of the most common forms of disability and diseases in the world (peptic ulcer disease, acid reflux disease, hepatitis, infections, various diarrheal diseases, constipation, and irritable bowel syndrome).

Therefore, a thorough understanding of the functions of the digestive system is essential for not only maintaining good health and nutrition but also for providing the most appropriate and effective treatment for its illnesses. In this regard our inadequate understanding of the digestive system is partly the cause of our ongoing struggle with many of the diseases. One example is IBD. Although its primary site is in the digestive tract, its effects can be systemic, involving the eyes, the skin, the musculoskeletal system, the immune system, nutrition, as well as psychological manifestations. This is, at least in part, due to the all-encompassing characteristic of the digestive system involving multiple organ systems in the body. As medical scientists make continued strides in their understanding of the body with the help of modern technology, better treatments, or perhaps even cures, for many of the diseases are anticipated.

CHAPTER 2

THE CAUSE OF INFLAMMATORY BOWEL DISEASE

Bret A. Lashner

SEARCHING FOR THE CAUSE

Finding the cause of inflammatory bowel disease (IBD) will lead to the cure through both treatment and prevention. Treatment of the causal agent should reduce inflammation and alleviate symptoms. Furthermore, preventing the causal agent from initiating inflammation in the bowel should decrease the occurrence of IBD in the general population. Searching for the cause of IBD is of paramount importance.

Epidemiology is defined as the study of factors that lead to disease. Since IBD does not occur evenly in all populations in the world, the study of the epidemiology of IBD can identify the reasons of this uneven distribution, which in turn could lead to important clues for finding the cause of IBD. For example, a cluster of IBD

Department of Gastroenterology, Cleveland Clinic Foundation,
Cleveland, Ohio 44195

cases among factory workers may point to an occupational exposure as a cause. Or, a sudden increase in IBD cases in a school could point to an infectious agent such as a virus as a cause. Or, an observation of the striking similarity of Crohn's disease (CD) occurrence rates over the last 50 years and cigarette smoking rates in the United States might suggest that a component of cigarette smoke is a causal factor for CD.

Classical epidemiology classifies disease occurrence by differences in person, place, and time. Classification by age, sex, race, physical activity, genetic markers, and socioeconomic status all are examples of "person variability." "Place variability" of disease identifies geographic similarities and occupational clustering. Also, changes in disease occurrence in migrating populations, or groups of people who move from a low-incidence IBD area to a high-incidence IBD area, can provide important clues as to the cause of IBD. "Time variability" examines changes in disease incidence with calendar year, seasonal variation, and certain age-related exposures such as cigarette smoking and medication use.

There are many holes in our knowledge of the epidemiology of IBD. Much information still needs to be collected and analyzed. However, promising leads exist and careful study of the person, place, and time variability of IBD is likely to point to the true cause or causes of IBD and the eventual cure through prevention and innovative treatments.

"PERSON" VARIABILITY OF IBD

IBD occurs most commonly among persons in the second and third decade of life (Fig. 1). There is a second, and much smaller, peak in the sixth decade. Males and females have a similar occurrence of IBD, but males have a 20% higher incidence of ulcerative colitis than females and females have a 20% higher incidence of CD than males. Are there hormonal causes for CD? Are there occupational risks for ulcerative colitis? More studies are needed to answer these questions.

IBD is very rare in African blacks whereas African-Americans have IBD incidence rates similar to American whites, suggesting an environmental, and not genetic, cause to IBD. On the other hand,

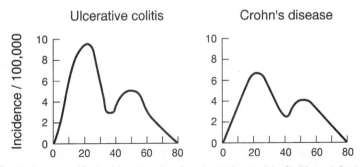

FIG. 1. Age-specific incidence rates for ulcerative colitis **(left)** and Crohn's disease **(right)** per 100,000 population. Note that each disease has a peak incidence in the second decade of life and a second smaller peak incidence in the fifth decade of life.

Ashkenazic Jews (Eastern European ancestry) in America have higher rates of IBD than Sephardic Jews (Spanish and North African ancestry) in America, suggesting a genetic predisposition.

IBD runs in families. Approximately 25% of IBD patients will have a family member (first cousin or closer relation) affected with IBD. Up to 1% of children of IBD patients will develop IBD over their lifetime. When IBD runs in families, there is an overwhelming likelihood for both affected family members to have the same type of IBD. Family members of CD patients have a higher likelihood of developing CD than ulcerative colitis, and family members of ulcerative colitis patients more often develop ulcerative colitis than CD.

Much research has been done to find the "IBD gene" or series of genes that lead to the uncontrolled inflammatory response of IBD. Indeed, there have been promising results in this field of study. Perinuclear antineutrophil cytoplasmic antibody (p-ANCA) is determined genetically and presents in up to 75% of ulcerative colitis patients. Only 5% to 10% of CD patients, a similar proportion to the general non-IBD population, are positive for p-ANCA. Whether or not p-ANCA-positive patients are more likely to respond to certain therapies, more likely to develop certain complications, or more likely to have p-ANCA-positive relatives who develop IBD in the future is of great clinical interest that needs to be answered.

Other genetically determined markers of IBD have been described and may hold clues to the causes of disease. Intestinal permeability, the ability of the intestine to allow large and potentially toxic compounds to enter the bloodstream, is increased in IBD. IBD patients have a "leaky" intestine that does not act as an effective barrier for toxic chemicals. Furthermore, certain unaffected relatives of IBD patients have abnormal intestinal permeability. Whether or not these are the relatives who will develop IBD in the future remains to be seen.

Genetic associations in IBD are only part of the answer. There are several "environmental" associations with IBD that are consistent and appear to be real. For example, IBD occurs more often in patients with a sedentary lifestyle—couch potatoes beware! IBD is more common in persons with higher incomes and in countries that are more developed. Cigarette smokers are more likely than non-smokers to develop CD. Curiously, cigarette smoking protects against the development of ulcerative colitis. In the person genetically predisposed to develop IBD, do these environmental factors determine the type of IBD that develops?

"PLACE" VARIABILITY OF IBD

Apparently, IBD occurs more commonly as one moves away from the equator. North America (excluding Latin America), Scandinavia, Northern Europe, Australia, and South Africa all have higher rates of IBD than the rest of the world (Fig. 2). Even in the United States, the northern tier of states has a higher rate of IBD. Notable exceptions are Florida and Arizona, states with large "snowbird" populations. Among differences in factors such as diet, lifestyle, and genetics, people in equatorial regions are exposed to more sunlight and consequently have higher levels of calcium and vitamin D than populations in higher latitudes. Could calcium supplementation protect against IBD? That is a question worthy of study.

Studies on migrant populations are the most important way to determine an "environmental" cause of disease. People who migrate from a low-IBD-risk country to a high-IBD-risk country tend to develop IBD at the rate of the high-IBD-risk country within one generation. Unfortunately, studies on migrant populations are rare and inconsistent. More of these important epidemiologic studies are needed. Urban centers have a higher rate of IBD than more rural

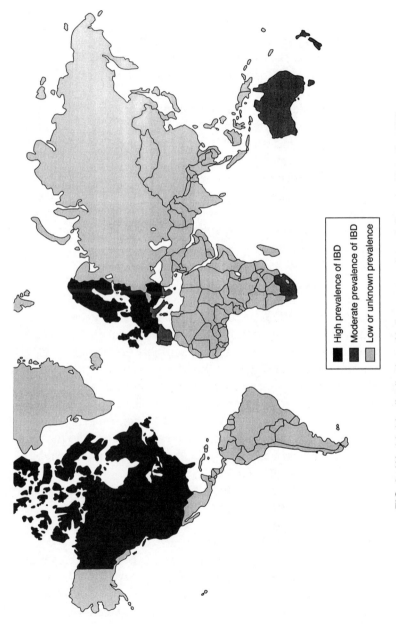

FIG. 2. Worldwide distribution of inflammatory bowel disease. Note that IBD tends to be more common as one moves further away from the equator in either a north or a south direction.

High prevalence of IBD

Moderate prevalence of IBD

Low or unknown prevalence

areas. Urban stress or urban pollution may have important causal roles that could be investigated.

Epidemiologists look for clustering of disease to try to identify an infectious organism as a cause of disease. Such clustering directly led to the identification of the bacteria responsible for Legionnaire's disease or the virus responsible for the AIDS epidemic. If IBD has an infectious cause, the organism has escaped detection to date. Classic patters of epidemic clustering and spread are not evident for IBD. Furthermore, extensive antibiotic use of many different formulations over the years has not lead to a decrease in IBD occurrence. Still, circumstantial evidence exists for *Mycobacterium paratuberculosis* (a bacterium related to the tuberculosis bacterium), *Paramyxovirus* (the measles virus), or *Entamoeba histolytica* (amoeba) to be potential causes of IBD. If these or other organisms are found to be associated with IBD, then the search for the proper antibiotic or vaccine will become paramount.

"TIME" VARIABILITY OF IBD

The occurrence of IBD is on the rise. In the United States over the last 40 years, rates of both ulcerative colitis and CD have gone up but the rise in the occurrence in CD has been most dramatic (Fig. 3). Genetic "drift" cannot account for this rapid change. Interestingly, this rise in CD occurrence closely parallels the increase in cigarette smoking rates in U.S. adults. Cigarette smokers have approximately 3 times the likelihood of developing CD than nonsmokers. There must be something in cigarette smoke that contributes to the development of CD. Everyone, but especially CD patients, must be strongly encouraged to quit smoking!

Cigarette smoking is an age- and era-related phenomenon. Cigarette smoking is out of fashion now and relatively less common in the "baby boom" generation. With a decrease in cigarette smoking rates in the United States in the last 5 years there has been a concomitant decrease in heart disease. It would be extremely interesting if CD posted a similar decline in the coming years. The effects of other age- and era-related environmental exposures, such as oral contraceptive use or being breast-fed as an infant, have enjoyed pop-

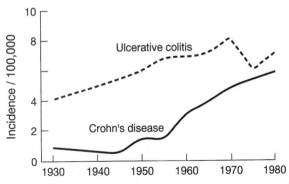

FIG. 3. Incidence rates per 100,000 population of ulcerative colitis and Crohn's disease from 1930 to 1980. Note that although the incidence of both ulcerative colitis and Crohn's disease has increased, the rise in the incidence of Crohn's has been dramatic.

ularity as potential causes of or protective mechanisms for IBD; however, studies have been weak and inconsistent.

Why does IBD more commonly exacerbate in the spring and fall? Why are nonsmokers more likely than smokers to develop ulcerative colitis? Why do children, a nonsmoking population, develop CD? Why do smokers in equatorial regions not develop CD? Perhaps the answer to these enigmas will shed light on the cause of IBD.

GENETICS VERSUS ENVIRONMENT

Is it nature or nurture? Is IBD in the genes or is it caused by environmental exposures? There is good evidence for both theories. A compromise theory for the cause of IBD is that a genetically predisposed individual will develop IBD if exposed to the critical environmental agent. Not much can be done to alter one's genetic make-up. Therefore, it is of crucial importance for epidemiologic investigation to continue to identify environmental, and hence treatable and preventable, causes of IBD. The identification of the critical environmental agents that cause IBD is sure to lead to recommendations to prevent high-risk exposures as well as to search for new and improved therapies.

CHAPTER 3

ULCERATIVE COLITIS

Richard P. Rood

Ulcerative colitis (UC) is an inflammatory disease of the large intestine, known as the colon, which is characterized by inflammation and ulceration of its innermost lining. In 50% of patients with UC, the disease affects only the lowest part of the colon, known as the rectum, and can be termed ulcerative proctitis. If the disease affects only the left side of the colon, it is called *limited* or *distal colitis*. If it involves the entire colon, it is termed *pancolitis* or *universal colitis*. Ulcerative colitis differs from Crohn's disease (CD), another inflammatory bowel disease (IBD). Ulcerative colitis affects only the colon. The inflammation is maximal in the rectum and extends up the colon in a continuous manner without any skip areas of normal intestine. Crohn's disease can affect any area of the gastrointestinal tract, including the small intestine, and have areas of normal intestine, so-called skip areas. Ulcerative colitis affects only the innermost lining of the colon, known as the mucosa, whereas CD can affect the entire thickness of the bowel wall. Ulcerative colitis and CD are different from, and should not be confused with, irritable bowel syndrome, also known as spastic colon. Irritable bowel syn-

Department of Medicine, Lake Hospital System, Willoughby, Ohio 44094, Division of Gastroenterology, Case Western Reserve University School of Medicine, Cleveland, Ohio 44132

drome is a noninflammatory motility disorder of the gastrointestinal tract. Irritable bowel syndrome bears no direct relationship to either UC or CD.

It is estimated that there are up to 1 million Americans with UC. The onset of the disease in the largest proportion of UC patients generally begins between the ages of 20 and 30 years, although it can occur in the mid-50s. The disease can occur at any age, is approximately 30% more common in females than males, and is also more common in Jews than non-Jews.

SYMPTOMS

The role of the colon in the body is to absorb fluid and electrolytes (salts) from the stool. Symptoms of UC can vary with both the location and severity of the disease. Symptoms of UC characteristically include diarrhea, rectal bleeding, and abdominal pain. Diarrhea might include both watery stool or more frequent soft stools, and can vary with both diet and disease activity. Patients might complain of spasm in the rectal area causing them to have frequent, small loose stools. As differs from patients with UC which involves the entire colon, patients with ulcerative proctitis may have constipation rather than diarrhea, as the majority of their colons are absorbing fluid and electrolytes properly and forming a solid stool. Rectal bleeding is common in patients with UC and generally occurs with increasing disease activity.

Abdominal pain is also common in patients with UC. The pain is characteristically crampy in nature and occurs usually in the lower abdomen, but can occur in any area of the abdomen. The pain is generally related to having a bowel movement, and either improves or is exacerbated by bowel movements. This pain is due to irritability and spasm of the colon because of the inflammation in the area. Finally, when UC is severe, the abdominal pain may also become severe, and marked abdominal distention may occur in association with a high fever. The abdominal pain can be accompanied by nausea, vomiting, and dehydration. These symptoms are characteristic of what is known as toxic megacolon, which is a severe complication of UC where the colon becomes markedly dilated and can perforate. This requires prompt medical attention.

Ulcerative colitis can also be associated with symptoms that are not specifically intestinal. These can include arthritis with pain and stiffness in the joints, skin lesions, and, in children, failure to grow properly especially when the disease is active.

DIAGNOSIS

The diagnosis of UC is based on the taking of a thorough clinical history of the symptoms described above. Initially, UC needs to be differentiated from infectious causes of diarrhea, whether or not blood is present. Other causes of diarrhea may be either bacterial, parasitic, or viral. It is important to know whether the patient has traveled to areas of the world where infectious diarrhea is common. In addition, patients who have been on antibiotics within the previous 6 months are at risk for developing a specific bacteria-induced diarrhea. It is also important to learn whether the patient has consumed any raw meats or shellfish that can harbor bacteria that can cause diarrhea. Finally, if multiple family members become ill with the same symptoms, it is more likely that the illness has an infectious cause. To confirm this, special stool cultures are ordered to identify the organism causing these symptoms.

Once infectious causes of diarrhea have been ruled out, the patient generally undergoes an examination of the colon by either sigmoidoscopy or colonoscopy. Flexible sigmoidoscopy involves the passage of a flexible instrument into the rectum and lower colon in order to see the extent and severity of the inflammation. The instrument has a light on the end of it; either the image is passed to the top of the scope to be examined by the physician or it is transmitted via a video system to a television monitor for viewing. Flexible sigmoidoscopy is used to examine the lowest 60 cm (2 feet) of the colon and is generally performed in a physician's office without sedation, as the procedure is fairly well tolerated. Colonoscopy is used to examine the entire colon and can be a more uncomfortable procedure. Patients are generally taken to an endoscopy facility and are sedated. Both flexible sigmoidoscopy and colonoscopy allow the physician to determine the quantity and position of the inflammatory changes. The physician may also biopsy the lining of the colon and send samples to a pathologist for further review.

The combination of flexible sigmoidoscopy, colonoscopy, and biopsy review can assist in the differential diagnosis of UC from other diseases of the colon. Ulcerative colitis is always worse in the rectum and follows in a continuous manner up the colon. CD has skip lesions, or normal areas, and granulomas, which are microscopic changes. Microscopic colitis appears grossly normal but has microscopic inflammation. Diverticular disease is characterized by diverticula, or pouches, along the side wall of the colon that can become inflamed or bleed. Other noninflammatory bleeding lesions of the colon include benign colon polyps and colon cancer.

MEDICAL TREATMENT

Currently, no medical cure for UC exists. However, effective medical treatment can suppress inflammation, permit healing of the colon, and relieve the symptoms of diarrhea, rectal bleeding, and abdominal pain associated with UC. Inflammatory cells and the bioactive chemicals produced by these cells in the lining of the colon cause the symptoms of UC. Therapy directed at these inflammatory cells and these chemicals can control the symptoms of this disease. Medications used in the treatment of IBD are reviewed completely in Chapter 10. Of the many medications used to treat IBD, three major classes of medications are used to treat UC. They are:

1. *Aminosalicylates.* These include aspirin-like medications such as sulfasalazine and 5-aminosalicylic acid (5-ASA, mesalamine, olsalazine). Sulfasalazine was the first of the agents developed originally as an antiinflammatory drug for arthritis. Taken orally, sulfasalazine is broken down in the intestine to its two ingredients, sulfapyridine and 5-ASA. Sulfapyridine is absorbed in the small bowel and excreted in the urine, and has little or no antiinflammatory activity. The active antiinflammatory substrate, 5-ASA, travels to the inner lining of the colon, acts on the inflammatory cells, and prevents the release of bioactive chemicals. Much of the side effects of sulfasalazine are attributed to sulfapyridine and not 5-ASA. New compounds, such as mesalamine and olsalazine, have been made to deliver

pure 5-ASA to the diseased colon and can be administered either orally or rectally. Controlled studies have clearly demonstrated that these agents are effective in the treatment of mild to moderate episodes of UC. Aminosalicylates are some of the few agents proven to maintain disease-free remission of UC.

2. *Corticosteroids.* These medications include prednisone, methylprednisolone, and budesonide, and can be given orally, rectally, or intravenously. Corticosteroids also suppress the inflammatory process in the colon and have a small direct antidiarrheal effect. These medications are used in moderate to severe cases of the disease and are effective in achieving remission of active UC.

3. *Immunomodulatory medicines.* These include azathioprine, 6-mercaptopurine (6-MP) (azathioprine's active byproduct), methotrexate, and cyclosporine, which inhibit the body's immune cells from interacting with the inflammatory process. These medications are administered orally, although methotrexate can be administered by intramuscular injection, and in patients with severe UC, cyclosporine can be administered intravenously. Azathioprine and 6-MP have been useful in reducing or eliminating the dependence on corticosteroids in some patients, and may be useful in maintaining remission. However, these two medications can take as long as 3 months to become effective. Studies are underway with methotrexate and cyclosporine, a powerful antirejection transplant medication. Currently, the definitive role for these two medications remains to be seen.

Symptomatic treatment not directed at the underlying inflammatory disease process is often effective in the management of UC patients. Avoidance of caffeine and lactose in patients with lactose intolerance can reduce diarrhea in some patients. In some cases, bulk-forming agents, such as Metamucil (Procter and Gamble, Cincinnati, OH) or Citrucel (SmithKline Beecham Consumer Healthcare, Pittsburgh, PA), can help decrease the volume of debilitating diarrhea. Antimotility agents, such as diphenoxylate (Lomotil, G.D. Searle and Co., Chicago, IL) and loperamide (Imodium, Janssen Pharmaeutical Inc., Titusville, NJ), can also be used to control the diarrhea of UC. However, caution should be taken using antimotility agents in patients with moderate to severe inflammatory disease. There is a risk of developing toxic megacolon, a life-threatening complication of UC.

SURGICAL TREATMENT

The only cure for UC is the surgical removal of the entire colon. This differs from CD, which can occur elsewhere in the gastrointestinal tract following the removal (resection) of the diseased segment. Surgery is recommended for those patients in which the disease is either not controllable medically or when complications of the disease occur. Traditional surgery involves removal of the entire colon and rectum and bringing the end of the remaining small bowel out through the skin of the abdominal wall forming a stoma, called an *ileostomy*. New surgical techniques have been developed to remove the colon, maintain bowel continuity and continence, and avoid an ileostomy. These techniques involve the creation of an internal pouch from a section of small intestine and the attachment of this pouch to the anal sphincter muscle area, maintaining bowel integrity and avoiding an external stoma or ileostomy. Further information regarding surgery and UC can be found in Chapter 11.

COMPLICATIONS

Intestinal Complications

Toxic Megacolon

Occasionally, UC progresses to fulminant colitis, where the colon loses its muscular tone and the its lumen becomes critically dilated. If the process is not reversed quickly, perforation will occur with an ensuing infection of the abdominal cavity, called *peritonitis*. Because of the risk of peritonitis, toxic megacolon is considered a medical-surgical emergency. While the majority of patients will require emergent surgery, the use of medications, such as cyclosporine, is being studied in the hope of avoiding surgery.

Colon Cancer

Ulcerative colitis patients have an increased risk of developing colon cancer. This risk can be as high as 3% to 5%, and increases with pancolitis and with the long-term duration of the disease. Colon cancer usually occurs as large bulky tumors in one's 50s and 60s. Colon cancer in UC patients generally occurs as a flat lesion and can be difficult to see in a colon that is markedly inflamed. Based on the increased incidence of cancer in UC patients who have had the disease for more than 8 years, it is recommended that patients be followed with surveillance colonoscopy approximately every year after that time to look for signs of pre-malignant changes, called *dysplasia.* Surveillance colonoscopy involves traditional colonoscopy with multiple biopsies throughout the colon to look for dysplasia. Dysplasia refers to changes in the cells of the colon, which behave more like tumor cells than regular colon cells. Once dysplasia is found and confirmed, colectomy is recommended, as colon cancer is likely to develop if it has not already.

Extraintestinal Complications

Extraintestinal (nonintestinal) complications of UC can occur in up to 45% of patients with UC. A more in-depth discussion of the complications of UC and CD can be found in Chapter 5. Complications involving blood, joints, skin, liver, eyes, and kidneys include the following:

1. *Anemia.* Patients with UC have chronic rectal bleeding. There is a constant loss of red blood cells and of the iron contained in them. Patients with active UC can develop iron deficiency anemia. This type of anemia corrects when iron stores are replenished either orally or intravenously. Patients on sulfasalazine can become folic acid–deficient. Sulfasalazine blocks the body's ability to absorb folic acid from food. Patients are often given supplemental folic acid to avoid this complication.
2. *Arthritis.* This includes diseases that can effect the joints, such as arthritis associated with IBD and ankylosing spondylitis. These two complications vary as to which joints are involved and whether the course of the arthritis mirrors the activity level of the underlying bowel disease.
3. *Skin.* Diseases can also effect the skin, causing the skin nodules of erythema nodosa and the skin ulcerations of pyoderma gangrenosa. Erythema nodosa can parallel the disease activity level of UC; pyoderma gangrenosa does not.

4. *Liver.* There are specific liver diseases associated with UC. The milder form is called pericholangitis, which involves inflammation around the small bile ducts that drain bile from the liver. The more severe and less frequent form is sclerosing cholangitis, which is characterized by both inflammation and scarring of the bile ducts. When the bile ducts become scarred, it can lead to chronic liver disease, cirrhosis, and liver failure, ultimately requiring a liver transplant. Sclerosing cholangitis is rare and treatments are being studied to slow the progression of this complication.

5. *Eyes.* Different sections of the eye can become inflamed causing uveitis and iritis. The symptoms include redness and pain around the eyes. These diseases respond to corticosteroid eye drops and require medical attention.

6. *Kidneys.* Since UC is a chronic diarrheal disease and patients are often dehydrated, their urine is more concentrated. Concentrated urine contains precipitating salts, which can form kidney stones. As with any other diarrheal illness, maintenance of proper fluid hydration is important.

PROGNOSIS

The course of the disease is dependent on many factors, including the disease severity (mild versus severe), extent (proctitis versus pancolitis), and associated intestinal and extraintestinal complications of the disease. Maintenance medication has been shown to significantly decrease the exacerbations of the disease. In between exacerbations, most patients feel well and are relatively free of symptoms. As discussed in Chapter 11, colectomy is necessary in approximately 20% to 25% of patients. The major incidence of requiring colectomy occurs in the first few years of the disease, and in children and adolescents because the disease can be more severe in these patients. In later years of the disease, the colectomy rate rises again as the risk of cancer increases. While UC is a serious chronic disease, it is not a fatal illness. Even though persons with UC may need to take regular medication and may occasionally need to be hospitalized, most continue to lead normal, useful, and productive lives.

CHAPTER 4

CROHN'S DISEASE

Burton I. Korelitz

HISTORICAL PERSPECTIVE

Why bother once again with history when patients demand fact and solution? Facts have been provided in a methodical and painstaking manner—many of them negative, requiring retreat to the last fork in the road, but also many positive, serving as stepping stones to the next bit of clarification. Why history? Because Crohn's disease (CD), despite the accumulated facts, remains a disease of unknown cause, and history taunts us with clues that have not yet been captured and dealt with. What are these clues?

1. The average age of onset is the teen years.
2. The younger the patient, the more virulent the course.
3. Despite the early description of regional ileitis by Crohn, Ginzburg, and Oppenheimer, there is now recognition that any segment of the bowel can be involved.
4. The onset of symptoms occurs only after the disease has become well established.
5. There are characteristic manifestations including diarrhea, perirectal fistulas, fistulas from the diseased bowel to adjoining

Department of Gastroenterology, Lenox Hill Hospital, New York, New York 10021; and Department of Medicine, New York University School of Medicine, New York, New York, 10016

    areas or other loops of bowel, strictures, skip areas, retarded growth and development, and a clear-cut family relationship in at least one third of cases.

6. No matter how severe the disease becomes, it usually remains localized to the segment of bowel where it was originally demonstrated. If, however, the bowel is resected or even transected, there is almost always extension of the disease proximally, usually at the line of anastomosis where the two healthy-appearing ends of bowel are sewn together.

7. When CD recurs after surgery, the form of recurrence mimics the original, i.e., with inflammation but no stricturing, with abscess and fistula formation but no stricturing, or with scarring and obstruction but no systemic signs of inflammation and no abscess or fistula.

8. Some cases respond adequately to drug preparations of 5-aminosalicylic acid (5-ASA), very similar to aspirin, whereas others do not.

9. The more severe cases respond dramatically to broad-spectrum immunosuppressives such as corticosteroids, and the underlying inflammation recurs as the medication is stopped or when the dose is reduced.

10. Immunosuppressive drugs such as oral 6-mercaptopurine (6-MP) and azathioprine are successful for chronic disease, and the intravenous immunosuppressive drug cyclosporine for severe disease. This may imply an immunologic defect that is being suppressed.

11. Antibiotics seem to work only in some cases. Does this imply an infectious agent or does the antibiotic work through some other route?

12. Despite all of these clues and everything we know, we still don't know why CD occurs in some people. Perhaps fresh minds—both knowledgeable physicians and untrained lay persons—will look at these clues now, 70 years later, and see what is being missed.

SIGNS, SYMPTOMS, AND DIAGNOSIS

The most characteristic symptoms either serve to make the diagnosis or lead to tests that will tell us what is happening.

1. There can be many causes of loose stools or watery diarrhea, but symptoms that persist for more than a few days warrant a diagnostic workup if one is not already underway. Stool studies for the culture of pathogenic bacteria, stool examination for parasites, and a *Clostridium difficile* test for patients whose onset of diarrhea followed an antibiotic regimen are essential. If negative, a workup is required, earlier in young people than in old.

2. A family history of CD or ulcerative colitis (UC) should provide a clue. So should abdominal cramps or pain. So should tenderness, particularly in the right lower quadrant of the abdomen. The sense of a mass in that area increases the likelihood of the diagnosis of CD.

3. The occurrence of an abscess or a fistula in or near the rectum, particularly in combination with the diarrhea or abdominal pain, increases the suspicion. Fistulas appearing on the abdominal wall or between the rectum and vagina are also characteristic of CD. The latter may be spontaneous or appear in the track of a scar resulting from a recent operation such as an appendectomy. The former manifests itself by passing of air through the vagina; then vaginal discharge; then even stool. Should a fistula extend from the bowel to urinary bladder, the symptoms will include air in the urine, signs of a urinary tract infection, or even the passage of stool in the urine.

4. The addition of anemia, fever, loss of appetite, and weight loss makes a diagnosis of CD still more likely and should lead to earlier diagnostic evaluation.

5. The next step will be influenced by the presumed location of the disease. Diarrhea, particularly when bloody, and lower abdominal pain suggest colonic involvement, whereas nausea, upper abdominal pain, and fever support small intestinal involvement. The source of the lower bowel syndrome will best be recognized by an endoscopy via the rectum. A flexible sigmoidoscopy serves to evaluate the rectum and the left colon and might lead to recognition of inflammation consistent with CD. Nevertheless, a full colonoscopy from the rectum to the ileum is preferred because CD of the colon while very active can spare the rectum and even the left colon. When inflamma-

tion is encountered there are features such as nodularity, superficial ulceration, and deep ulceration that are characteristic of CD. So are asymmetric involvement, skip areas, areas of exudate (pus), and strictures. Biopsies can be suggestive of CD but are not confirmatory without recognition of microscopic lesions called granulomas or microgranulomas by the pathologist. The most distal segment of the small bowel, known as the terminal ileum, enters the colon at the cecum. Since the terminal ileum is usually involved if the right side of the colon is involved, an attempt to enter this segment should be tried with the colonoscope. If, however, the terminal ileum is involved, it is usually narrowed or even strictured and such a maneuver is not possible.

6. If the symptoms suggest upper GI or small bowel involvement, then barium contrast x-rays are appropriate (the GI/small bowel x-ray series). This can serve to outline characteristic lesions of CD including ulcerations, nodules, strictures, fistulas, and inflammatory masses. Since the most common distribution of CD is a combination of ileum and colon, ideally a diagnostic evaluation for CD should include both a colonoscopy and the GI/small bowel x-rays.

7. A barium enema x-ray examination is no longer indicated as often as a colonoscopy for evaluation. Nevertheless, this x-ray examination remains better than the endoscopy for demonstrating fistulas entering the colon, for outlining strictures, and for refluxing barium into the terminal ileum when examination of that segment cannot be accomplished by the endoscopy.

8. Examination of the rectum is essential in establishing a diagnosis of CD. On inspection the examiner may confront abscesses or pus being expressed via fistulas. The anus might be the site of waxy-appearing skin tabs, which are often called hemorrhoids but are actually hypertrophied inflamed tissue diagnostic of CD and referred to as elephant ears. On introduction of the finger into the rectum other characteristic features of CD may be encountered such as nodules, polyps, and strictures.

9. Abdominal masses felt on examination can be further evaluated by computed tomographic (CT) scans and sonograms. These diagnostic imaging examinations often outline a mass or dis-

close an abscess or fistula not appreciated by conventional barium x-rays.

10. A diagnosis of obstruction is often suspected by physical examination but better established by plain x-rays of the abdomen
taken in the lying and erect positions.

11. Crohn's disease may be manifest in organ systems other than the
bowel. These extraintestinal manifestations include skin lesions
(pyoderma gangrenosum and erythrema nodosum), mouth and
lip lesions (aphthous ulcers), eye lesions (uveitis), liver abnormalities, joint inflammations (arthritis), urinary tract stones,
gallstones, and syndromes due to malabsorption of various
ingredients of the diet. Most of these systemic or extraintestinal
manifestations parallel the severity of the CD in the bowel, but
others, characterized by sacroilitis (arthritis of the spine), primary sclerosing cholangitis (narrowing of the bile ducts), and
pyoderma gangrenosum, may not.

DIFFERENTIAL DIAGNOSIS

Once a negative stool evaluation for the cause of diarrhea has led
to a diagnostic workup and the physical examination and laboratory
tests suggest no other diagnoses, the contribution of colonoscopy
and GI/small bowel x-rays almost always clarify the diagnosis of CD
and also define the extent of involvement in the GI tract.

One major exception to this rule is the inflammatory process limited to the colon and not involving the small bowel, which would
have supported the diagnosis of CD.

1. A colitis due to a variety of causes may mimic CD of the colon
(Crohn's colitis). If other characteristic features of CD are present, then it is much easier to differentiate from other forms of
colitis.
    a. *Infectious*, most commonly *Salmonella, Shigella, E. coli,
    Cryptosporidium*, all found by stool culture.
    b. *Parasitic*, most commonly amebic, found by stool examina-
    tion.
    c. *Pseudomembranous*, usually caused by antibiotics, suspected
    on sigmoidoscopy, and caused by the *C. difficile* bacteria.

d. *Ischemic,* due to vascular insufficiency. These are seen mostly in elderly patients but also in young patients, due to various forms of bowel twisting or vascular complications, and are often recognized by endoscopy, biopsy, and/or various x-rays techniques.

e. *Radiation colitis* follows radiation treatment of cancer of the uterus, ovary, or prostate, suspected by history and recognized by endoscopy and biopsies.

f. *Cytomegalovirus* (CMV) occurring mostly in immunocompromised patients and recognized by biopsies.

g. *Diversion colitis,* following diversion of the fecal stream by ileostomy or colostomy, and recognized by history and its reversal by reanastamosis. This presents a particular problem in patients with CD who have had diversion surgery but the rectum had earlier been spared, raising the question of whether to resect the rectum or perform reanastamosis.

2. The differential diagnosis of CD from UC is a problem in approximately 7% of patients with colitis limited to the left colon and including the rectum. This is referred to as an indeterminate colitis. Unfortunately biopsies show non-specific features of inflammation and not the granuloma or deep involvement of the colonic wall characteristic of CD. When the colon is resected because of disease severity without resolution of the differential diagnosis, proof of the previous diagnosis having been CD is often first established by recurrent ileitis in the ileostomy or in the ileoanal pouch, both established with the conviction that the diagnosis at the time of resection was UC.

3. In the practice of a proctologist the fistula-in-ano is a common finding and unassociated with CD in most cases. Nevertheless, and particularly when the fistula is multiple or otherwise complex, a search for CD in the bowel should be undertaken.

4. A still common manner of presentation of CD is right lower quadrant abdominal pain and tenderness suggesting appendicitis. A complete history supplemented by x-ray imaging might clarify the diagnosis. Nevertheless, exploratory surgery is often required to confirm appendicitis and remove the appendix before it becomes perforated. This approach is usually justified and safe as opposed to perforated appendicitis with peritonitis.

A problem arises when the diagnosis of ileitis is then recognized and the surgeon chooses to perform a resection. This means that the patient is immediately subjected to extension of the ileitis proximally without ever having had the opportunity for drug therapy. Ideally, for a nonperforated ileitis found at exploration for probable appendicitis, the appendix should be removed if the adjoining cecum is not involved but not removed if the adjoining cecum is involved. The abdomen should then be closed without resection of the ileitis and a gastroenterologist should then be called in consultation for further management of the active ileitis.

COMPLICATIONS OF CROHN'S DISEASE

The term "complication" is fine for purposes of management but "progression of severity" would probably be a more appropriate term. Furthermore, many complications of CD can be traced to the medical and surgical therapy, use of which nevertheless statistically favors a better outcome than nonuse of these modalities.

1. *Obstruction.* This term almost always refers to small bowel obstruction based on the facts that the most distal small bowel (terminal ileum), with or without involvement of the adjoining colon, is the most common segment of distribution of CD and that the small bowel is much narrower than the large bowel to begin with. Due to progressive inflammation and scarring in the small bowel, the lumen (or space) becomes progressively smaller and finally neither food nor gas can pass it. Colonic obstruction can also occur, particularly at the sites of stricture or giant inflammatory polyps, but this is much less common. Patients with CD have a definite advantage by chewing their food well so that a bolus of food is less likely to impact in the narrowed lumen and cause a still earlier obstruction than might otherwise have been the case. The most effective management of small bowel obstruction involves the passage of a small bowel tube, which is then attached to suction for decompression. The addition of intravenous steroids to reduce the inflammation in the small bowel (or colon) will hasten the opening of the lumen and relief of the obstruction. These maneuvers

require hospitalization. In some cases the use of oral steroids along with the elimination of all other oral feedings will be satisfactory. The choice should be based on the keen judgment of the managing gastroenterologist.

Bowel obstruction can be recognized by the clinical history in the setting of known CD and confirmed by physical examination and plain x-rays of the abdomen that reveal levels of air above fluid. Relief occurs first with the passage of air and then fluid by rectum will decrease in abdominal distention. At the right time, the patient may be started on clear fluids by mouth and then the tube may be withdrawn.

Chronic recurrent obstruction might very well require surgery, preferably on an elective basis. In some cases, resection of the obstructing segment is indicated, but when the obstructing segment is very short, a procedure called stricturolplasty might be sufficient. In some cases of extensive CD with multiple sites of obstruction, combinations of these two types of procedures are warranted.

2. *Abscesses and fistulas.* These complications too represent a progression of the CD process. They are considered together because it is the breakdown of the abscess that creates the fistula, which then drains to the skin or connects to another organ or another loop of bowel. The most common fistulas are perirectal, intrarectal, rectovaginal, ileoileal, ileocolic (especially to the sigmoid colon), ileovesical (the urinary bladder), and from the ileum or colon into the mesenteries which encompass the bowel.

As is the case with obstruction, infrequently should a fistula warrant surgical resection of the underlying bowel. In most cases the fistula will be eliminated or at least improved with immunosuppressive drugs used to treat the underlying CD. In the case of a perirectal abscess, surgical drainage or eradication is sometimes necessary to relieve pain or chronic distress. This maneuver might convert the abscess to a fistula, but it serves to buy time for treatment with immunosuppressive drugs to be successful. Small abscesses within intraabdominal masses will respond to treatment of the underlying bowel disease with intravenous steroids, supplemented by antibiotics. Larger abscesses, as recognized by x-ray imaging, may require evacuation by a needle administered by an interventional radiologist or, less often, open drainage performed by the surgeon.

3. *Malabsorption.* When CD involves large areas of small bowel, there may be interference with the absorption of normal food-stuffs. This is more common in children with CD where an extra demand for calories is dictated by growth and metabolism. In addition to optimum treatment of the underlying CD, food supplementation with proteins absorbed high in the bowel and even total parenteral nutrition (intravenous) are warranted.

4. *Extraintestinal manifestations* will be covered in Chapter 5.

5. *Premalignant changes* in the bowel and cancer of both the colon and small bowel will also be covered in Chapter 5. The ultimate risk of cancer in CD influences the management of other complications, particularly in the presence of strictures.

6. *Toxic megacolon.* Dilatation of the colon signifies that inflammation has spread throughout the wall and perforation is likely if not prevented. This is characteristic of severe UC but can occur in severe CD of the colon also. The earlier it is treated, the better the chance of a favorable response. It requires the stopping of oral feedings, small bowel tube decompression, intravenous steroids and antibiotics, and turning the patient from side to side to mobilize air and fluid. If there is no response within 3 to 5 days, ileostomy and colectomy are indicated. In most cases, the patient needs to be followed closely with physical examination and plain x-rays of the abdomen.

7. *Free perforation of the colon or small bowel* occurs rarely in CD. More often the sequence will be penetration, abscess formation, and a tender mass. Nevertheless, free perforation can occur and recognition of free air in the abdominal cavity should lead to immediate surgery.

MANAGEMENT

When ileitis was recognized as a distinct entity by Crohn, Ginzburg, and Oppenheimer, no effective drugs were available for treatment. Most of the innovations in management were reported by surgeons, and in fact patients were dramatically relieved by resection or bypass operations. They returned to the surgeon when the recurrence occurred for still another resection. Many such patients ended up with short bowel syndromes and malabsorption as well as recurrent ileitis.

With the introduction of sulfasalazine (Azulfidine, Pharmacia and Upjohn, Kalamazoo, MI) in Sweden, there was finally a drug that was effective against UC. It did work for CD of the colon but only in a few cases of ileitis. In the early 1950s corticosteroids and adrenocorticotropic hormone (ACTH) were discovered; remissions were initially dramatic and gastroenterologists were once again managing patients with CD. The following are the drugs in current use along with their indications, complications, and justifications for management. With appropriate use of these drugs, the number of patients requiring surgery has been markedly reduced. Nevertheless, the availability of surgeons and innovative surgical techniques remains essential for total management of patients with CD.

1. *Corticosteroids and ACTH* have led to more dramatic remissions of CD than ever observed. Because of the initial success of these drugs the motivation for research into new drug therapies was postponed. Within a few years, however, it became clear that the favorable results against CD were transient, that symptoms returned when the drugs were stopped and in many cases even when the dose was reduced, that the drugs caused a high degree of toxicity in proportion to dose and the amount of time that they were used. Furthermore, the steroids had no maintenance value once a remission was achieved.

   It is therefore now accepted that steroids [intravenous (IV) hydrocortisone, IV ACTH, IV prednisolone, oral prednisone] are acute phase drugs and serve to bring patients with CD into remission. They should serve to buy time to introduce more slowly acting drugs that are also effective, are less toxic, and maintain the remission.

   A newer steroid (budesonide, Astra, Sweden) which results in less toxicity than prednisone has been shown to be effective in the treatment of CD. While its therapeutic results are slightly less than those of prednisone, the minimal toxicity permits continuation for a longer time. Although it cannot be considered a maintenance drug, the lack of toxicity might serve to buy a longer period of time to maintain the asymptomatic state for the maintenance drugs to be effective.

2. *Sulfasalazine* has a small role in CD. The sulfa component of the drug is responsible for many toxic side actions while merely acting as a carrier to escort the other part of the drug, 5-ASA, through the small intestine until it is released by bacterial cleavage in the colon. The drug has had a role in CD but mostly when there is colonic involvement.

3. *5-ASA* is the active ingredient of sulfasalazine and in the last decade has been manufactured by four different drug companies in the United States in forms to be released at various sites of inflammation without the need for a sulfa carrier. These are Dipentum (Pharmacia and Upjohn, Kalamazoo, MI), Asacol (Procter and Gamble, Cincinnati, OH), Pentasa (Hoechst, Marion Roussel, Kansas City, MO), and Rowasa (Solvay Pharmaceuticals, Inc., Marietta, GA). Controlled trials have shown that these drugs are effective in controlling UC. Surprisingly, it was soon recognized that Asacol and Pentasa were also released in the small bowel and therefore could and did have a role in treatment of CD. Dipentum is not released until it reaches the colon and Rowasa (enemas and suppositories) are effective in proctitis. Dipentum and Rowasa have little or no role in the treatment of CD. Asacol, which is released in the distal small bowel, is effective for ileitis and Crohn's colitis. Pentasa may be released in the proximal segments of the small bowel and even at the level of the stomach; this drug would then be choice for extensive small bowel CD and CD of the stomach. Toxicity due to 5-ASA products is minimal. Dipentum can cause diarrhea. The others may be responsible to allergic reactions similar to those caused by aspirin where the formulation is similar. Some allergic reactions occur with one drug such as Asacol but not with Pentasa, suggesting that the coating of the drug may be more responsible for the allergic reaction than the drug itself. Infrequent inflammation of the lung and kidney have been reported. Alopecia (loss of hair) is fairly common wtih Asacol. All complications have been reversible on stopping the drug.

4. *6-MP* and azathioprine (the oral immunosuppressives) were introduced by Hitchings and Elion to prevent the rejection of

transplanted organs, whereupon they received the Nobel Prize. When CD (and UC) were considered autoimmune diseases, these drugs were submitted to trials. 6-MP proved to be effective in two thirds of cases of CD, serving to eliminate the need for steroids. They also served to close fistulas, the first drugs observed to accomplish this goal.

6-MP and azathioprine proved to be slow in their action taking from 3 to 6 months to be effective and meanwhile requiring reintroduction of steroids in some cases to buy that time. Toxicity due to the drugs occurs infrequently, usually within the first 3 weeks of treatment in the forms of allergic reactions, pancreatitis, and hepatitis, all of which are reversible on stopping the drug. The drugs can and often do lower the white blood count and sometimes the platelets. The problem has been modified by careful monitoring of the blood counts. Nevertheless, monitoring is an inconvenience for some.

There has also been a fear than 6-MP and azathioprine carry a permissive influence on the development of tumors. This has not been substantiated by long-term studies of toxicity where a variety of neoplasms have occurred in no greater incidence than the CD population in general. Even lymphomas have occurred only rarely and the oral immunosuppressives could not be blamed with the exception of two brain lymphomas that otherwise have been reported only in transplant cases. 6-MP and azathioprine have been the first drugs shown to have maintenance value in CD and to prevent recurrence after remission and surgical resection.

5. *Cyclosporine.* This immunosuppressive drug replaced Imuran as that most commonly use to prevent rejection after transplant surgery. Logically it was tried for CD as well. Trials of oral cyclosporine have demonstrated success in cases of CD but the overall results have been modest, perhaps due to inconsistency of absorption by the oral route. Using the drug intravenously has led to reversal of severe UC within 2 weeks in many cases, but with substitution of the oral cyclosporine the remission may be brief and the patients still require colectomy. Intravenous Cyclosporine has also been tried for complex fistulas of CD with impressive results. Again there is reversal when the drug is switched from the intravenous to the oral route. Initiation of oral

6-MP or azathioprine after fast remission with intravenous cyclosporine is being tried and shows more promise for maintenance than oral cyclosporine.

Just as cyclosporine has been tried for CD, the drug currently favored by transplant surgeons to prevent rejection, tacrolimus (Prograf, Fujisawa USA Inc., Deerfield IL), might also prove to have a role.

6. *Antibiotics*. There are patients with CD who seem to respond to choice antibiotics as well as to other drugs. These results have been inconsistent and the number of control trials have been few. Antibiotics have a supplementary role in the presence of infectious complications such as perirectal abscesses and a primary role in the treatment of toxic megacolon. Metronidazole (Flagyl, Searle) has a modest effect on the bowel manifestations of CD, but it has been effective against perirectal abscesses. Unfortunately, it requires a large dose, which often results in a peripheral neuritis. When the dose is reduced or the drug is stopped the perirectal disease returns.

7. *Methotrexate* (Lederle Laboratories, Pearl River, NY) has been administered intramuscularly with success in patients with CD. Its favorable results are modified when the drug is changed to the oral route. Because of side actions and limited effectiveness, its trial has been favored for those failing or allergic to 6-MP or azathioprine.

8. *Monoclonal antibodies*. The best example of this category of drug is anti-TNF, a drug which interferes with one of the known mediators of inflammation in UC called tumor necrosis factor. Studies have proven its effectiveness in CD as it is administered intravenously.

Many of the disclosures in the laboratory have been pursued by seeking the mechanism by which the drugs that we use have achieved success. Patients with CD should be encouraged by the success of our current drug armamentarium and its influence on the volume of basic research currently being performed.

SUGGESTED READING

Prantera C, Korelitz BI. *Crohn's disease*. New York: Marcel Dekker, 1996.

CHAPTER 5

EXTRAINTESTINAL COMPLICATIONS AND ASSOCIATED PROBLEMS OF INFLAMMATORY BOWEL DISEASE

Joel B. Levine and *Bernard Levin

*Department of Medicine, University of Connecticut School of Medicine, Farmington, Connecticut 06030, and *Division of Cancer Prevention, Department of Gastrointestinal Oncology and Digestive Diseases, University of Texas M.D. Anderson Cancer Center, Houston, Texas 77030*

PART A: EXTRAINTESTINAL COMPLICATIONS

Setting the Stage

On the battlefields of the First World War, French soldiers, stricken with dysentery (bloody diarrhea), unexpectedly complained of eye and/or joint symptoms during the time of their intestinal illness. Though unsure of the reason, physicians carefully recorded their findings hoping that the future would validate and explain these intriguing findings. In the 1930s, as ulcerative colitis (UC) was being intensively studied, another observation, i.e., an increase in the number of blood clots in those inflammatory bowel disease (IBD) patients with the most active symptoms, added to the impression that the intestinal process could be accompanied by a broader range of problems in other parts of the body. Over the next few decades, a recognizable cluster of recurring symptoms involving the eye, joints, and skin was frequently reported and became part of the clinical language. In the Indonesian Wyang or puppet theater, the play is presented by the shadows cast by unseen puppets held by the hidden puppeteer. The meaning of the play is felt to be best learned by the study of these shadows. So too are the extraintestinal events in IBD capable of illuminating new principles that influence the development and clinical course of these diseases.

At the heart of our changing knowledge is an important concept: The intestine is normally a barrier to the outside world, carefully regulating responses to a vast array of food as well as bacterial and viral proteins presented to it from earliest development and throughout life. By doing this, nature seeks a proper balance: selectively sampling proteins, ignoring those that will not do the body harm, but rejecting, through the process of inflammation, those whose successful penetration of this barrier could cause injury and illness. For reasons that are now just becoming more clear, this biological economy falters in IBD. The normally closely controlled inflammation reaction becomes overactive and less well regulated, more and more proteins cross into the intestinal lining further stimulating inflammatory responses, the tissue is injured and clinical symptoms and illness appear. As this cascade becomes chronic, an inability to restore the original protective properties of the intestinal surface leads to poor healing and an altered effort to repair that produces scarring and an eventual compromise of normal function.

This sustained inflammatory response activates an increasingly larger number of the body's white blood cells to produce chemicals (cytokines) that draw even more cells from the bloodstream to the area of inflammation. In fact, the blood vessels within the area of inflammation are themselves similarly altered, becoming two-way doors: accelerating the entrance of inflammatory cells and permitting the exit of proinflammatory products into the bloodstream. Inflammation in IBD is thereby transported to other areas of the body and consequently converts what was once a local response to a general and more extensive illness. When these proinflammatory materials are in the circulation, they find a receptive welcome at locations that can be recruited into the inflammatory reaction. Some joints, for example, have fluid-filled spaces that are lined with tissues containing many small blood vessels that permit both white blood cells and mediators to pass into the joint space fluid. Once present, the mediators overcome the fluid's natural resistance and initiate a response that produces the symptoms of hot, swollen, and painful joints.

Joints and the Skeleton

Although intestinal inflammation is present in all patients with IBD, not all develop extraintestinal features. In fact, only about 1 in 5 get any kind of joint or skeletal complaint and these patients are more likely to have disease involving the colon rather than the small intestine. Thus, joint problems are more common in those with UC or when Crohn's disease (CD) involves the large bowel. Furthermore, since the cause of the joint problems relates to the presence of intestinal inflammation, it is common to experience an increase in joint symptoms when the gut disease is itself more active. This is already known to many as the complaint of a stiff, painful, and swollen knee may precede the onset of more obvious intestinal problems. Even a level of inflammation sufficient to activate key white blood cells but not as enough to produce abdominal pain, diarrhea, or bleeding can cause the joints to make themselves known to you.

In children, for example, an arthritis-like picture may start long before anyone has suspected an underlying IBD. In any IBD patient, when the joints become active, it is usually the large joints, particularly knees, ankles, hips, and shoulders, that dominate the clinical picture. Small joint problems, i.e., the fingers and toes, so common in other conditions, are less likely to have any relation to the state of activity of the intestinal disease.

When the larger joints become active, it is often quite dramatic; they swell quickly and are quite tender. If the gut is active or becomes more active soon after the joints flare, the standard treatments of the active intestinal inflammation (sulfasalazine, 5-aminosalicylate, or steroids) are sufficient to reduce both sources of distress, i.e., as the colitis or small bowel inflammation becomes less active, the joints will usually follow. Patients learn to read the signals when their joints become involved and may start to treat their colitis/ileitis even before a change in the number of bowel movements or the presence of blood is upon them. It is important to remember that, for the most part, these affected joints do not develop a chronic injury. Patients should look at these problems as having a different impact from the cumulative damage seen in the more common disorders of osteoarthritis and rheumatoid arthritis. Certainly, any individual patient can have more than one disease but, in general, the joints in IBD patients retain the capacity to return to normal when the intestinal activity subsides. Only about 10% of those with joint symptoms develop and evolve any chronic joint damage, but if your complaints seem to stay around after the gut has quieted down, bring this to the attention of your physician.

It remains of great interest as to why only a small percentage of patients with IBD get joint problems. It is increasingly clear that among patients with UC or CD there are subtle individual differences that influence the course and consequence of these diseases. Many of these differences are guided by genetic (inheritance) factors and modified by various environmental pressures. One such factor is the differing ability of an individual patient's immune system to recognize and respond to specific bacterial species in the gut; some people can recognize a given type of germ and some cannot. This recognition uses a lock-and-key type of mechanism, with the number and shape of the locks determined by genes. Broadly speaking, those IBD patients who develop joint problems have specific locks that can be opened by certain keys (specific bacterial proteins) and by so doing uniquely activate an inflammatory response. Additionally, some keys may resemble, at least in part, a protein used in our own tissues. Thus a reaction triggered by a foreign key could invoke a response to the body's own structure. This is a basis for developing an autoimmune response. For example, patients with IBD and arthritis can develop antibodies against their own cartilage or collagen, the building blocks that comprise the joint architecture.

A word of caution to those who develop these joint symptoms: Do not reach for the usual antiinflammatory drugs of the nonsteroidal type, e.g., Advil, Motrin, Alleve, and the like. Although these are frequently helpful in reducing joint inflammation, their use in patients with IBD can be associated with a flare of the disease. In some difficult joint cases, your physician may inject steroids into the joint space to reduce inflammation but, in general, with successful treatment of the intestine, the joint symptoms will subside.

The Spine

Just as the large joints may be involved when the intestine is inflamed, the spine can become a source of discomfort (spondylitis). If one looks with sensitive imaging methods, the low back (the sacroiliac joint) may show inflammatory changes even if clinical complaints are not yet present. In those who eventually develop low-back-related symptoms, they are characteristically described: low back pain with morning stiffness, relieved by exercise, and often blamed on the mattress, lack of exercise, or poor posture.

When back problems occur, there may be changes in the spine and along its supporting ligaments, a loss of flexibility, and, over time, a decrease in chest expansion. In the very late stages, the upper or cervical spine can develop nerve problems not unlike those that occur in patients with "pinched nerve." It is important for your doctor to be aware of these skeletal problems and to examine you at regular intervals. If any symptoms occur, then a program of increased exercise, especially swimming and deep breathing exercises, will be helpful in keeping good function and minimizing disability. Remember that these changes, like those in the smaller joints, may occur when the intestine is quite silent but still driven by microscopic inflammation and cell activation.

Both patient and physician should also keep a watchful eye on the risks for bone thinning. This change, called osteopenia, was once thought to be primarily related to long-term or high-dose steroid exposure; however, it is now clear that the inflammatory process can alter bone metabolism, making it less likely that new bone will be formed and well mineralized. The degree of bone thinning can be quite substantial, especially in young people, and periodic measurements of bone density are well advised. Though progress has been made in keeping bones stronger, good control of the inflammation itself seems very important as the best primary protection.

The Eyes

Though it seems to bear little obvious similarity, the structure of the eye, with its large number of small blood vessels and fluid filled chamber is, like the joint, prepared to become involved in the extraintestinal events in IBD. There are several layers of these blood vessel–rich linings and depending on which layer is inflamed, different clinical symptoms will appear. The most common complaint is a red but not painful eye as the episclera becomes inflamed (episcleritis). This is often at the time of increased clinical bowel activity and subsides as the gut improves with therapy. If the uvea, a deeper layer, becomes involved, it is often in tune with joint and skin changes and presents with a painful eye (usually one side) with mild blurring but without marked changes in visual acuity (uveitis). On occasion, the layers involving the retina can be affected and significant changes in vision may occur. As with the joint, the eye changes can appear when the bowel is inflamed but the patient is not, i.e., when gut symptoms are minimal. Asymptomatic (silent) uveal changes can be detected and are important; if left untreated they can lead to a pattern of scarring that can produce glaucoma and cataracts. It is important, therefore, for IBD patients to have frequent eye examinations and especially if there are visible changes or symptoms. For the most part, the resolution of the gastrointestinal symptoms will be accompanied by improvement in the eye findings. However, occasionally the eye can progress even after the intestinal complaints have resolved, so that persisting symptoms should warrant physician attention.

The Skin

The skin may also reflect the events taking place in the intestine, and, as with the joint and the eye, provide a clue as to the degree of intestinal inflammation. The most common change is called erythema nodosum, which occurs in about the same numbers of patients as the complications already discussed. It often appears early in the course of IBD and, in almost 80% of cases, in the company of some form of joint inflammation. The patient will notice tender bumps, often on both legs, that may precede, by a varying period of time, a change in the bowel symptoms. Erythema nodosum is also seen in other conditions and may reflect the impact of cytokines crossing into the bloodstream. There is experimental evidence that if specific cytokines are injected directly under the skin, an erythema nodosum-like change can occur in some patients. Another skin response, often looked to with greater concern, may arise and seem indifferent to the state of IBD clinical activity or even to the success of IBD therapy. It is called pyoderma gangrenosum and may also reflect local response to increased amounts of proinflammatory chemicals. Pyoderma, although it means "pus under the skin," is mislabeled because, despite its appearance, it is not infected but shows intense injury to small blood vessels and their lining cells. Pyoderma is usually quite hard to treat and conventional therapies, even steroids, are not predictably or easily successful. Recently, the use of high oxygen content air (hyperbaric oxygen), not unlike what deep sea divers use when coming up from a deep dive, has shown promise though the therapy takes many sessions and a long time to show effect.

There are many other skin changes in IBD, many of which are even less well understood that those that we have discussed. CD, for example, may be associated with chancre sore–like ulcers of the mouth lining, some of which actually show a pathologic picture that strongly resembles the Crohn's injury seen in the intestine. Cracks in the corners of the mouth (cheilosis), splitting lips (fissuring), or even just reddening of the skin around the lips can be signs of the underlying intestinal process. For many of these skin changes there are no specific therapies available. Varied combinations of locally applied antibiotics, with or without steroids, vitamin E, or just the basics of good skin care are used with varying success. In general, the consulting advice of a dermatologist (skin specialist) is helpful if these changes have occurred or even if there is only the beginning of the suggestion of skin involvement.

A Wider Perspective

If you were to spend time looking through the medical literature, you would find evidence for changes for selected patients in almost every organ or body system. As noted previously, there is an increased risk for blood clots during the active intestinal inflammation due to an increase in inflammatory cell chemicals that promote clotting. The risk usually decreases with successful therapy of IBD but may persist in those with CD who smoke.

It is worth appreciating that the liver can be indirectly involved in IBD through an inflammation of its bile ducts, the tubes that carry bile from the liver to the gallbladder and the intestine. This occurs mainly in patients with UC and can result in scarring, obstruction, and infection of these tubes, producing fever and even jaundice (yellowing of the skin). This association is an important one, however, as the bile duct disease can be present before any clinical symptoms appear and progress despite effective therapy of the bowel, including colectomy. This inflammation, called sclerosing cholangitis, may be linked to IBD through specific genetic factors that are present in only a portion of the total number of UC cases. It is important for the doctor to periodically check liver function by blood tests and even to test for the genetic marker.

As with the liver, the kidneys may be effected by changes to the body brought about by the overall illness burden in IBD rather than by direct inflammation. This is most true for the risk for kidney stone formation, which is especially high in patients with disease, or absence, of the last part of the small intestine (the ileum). This leads to an increased urinary passage of stone-forming mineral crystals, particularly oxalate. Avoiding foods rich in oxalate, e.g., spinach, beets, turnips, tea, and cola, and ingesting sufficient oral fluids to prevent any dehydration can be very effective in preventing this complication. In addition, as the ureter (the tube that goes from the kidney to the bladder) may cross very near to the right colon or ileum, CD can lead, via bowel inflammation or scar formation, to obstruction and risk of infection to the kidney.

Summary

This review should not cause patients to become overly concerned that their disease will become more complicated or have certain effects on other parts of the body. Only a minority of all IBD patients have any problems at all and the most common are often successfully controlled when the bowel is brought to remission. It is important, however, for both the doctor and the patient to be aware that IBD can involve these distant areas so that any unusual symptoms can be quickly and accurately identified.

PART B: ASSOCIATED PROBLEMS

Cancer (Including Dysplasia and Surveillance)

Cancer of the gastrointestinal tract can arise as a rare complication of both longstanding CD and UC. Although malignancies of the small intestine have been described in association with CD, the remainder of this discussion will be confined to malignancies that arise in the large bowel (colon and rectum). Although fewer than 1% of all colorectal cancers arise in the setting of chronic IBD, the risk of developing a large bowel tumor is still a source of much concern for patients and their physicians.

Ulcerative Colitis

Risk

The first report in the medical literature of large bowel cancer occurring in the presence of UC occurred approximately 70 years ago. Over the past seven decades, improved statistical methodology has been developed that permits a more accurate risk assessment to be carried out. We can now conclude that after 25 years of symptoms of chronic UC, the risk of developing colorectal cancer is approximately 10% (1,2).

Risk Factors

1. *Extent of colonic involvement.* The risk for colorectal cancer is largely confined to those individuals in whom most of the colon at sometime has been involved by inflammation (2). The risk begins to arise above that of the general population after approximately 8 to 10 years of disease. Although patients with predominantly left-sided involvement only are also at risk of developing cancer, those whose involvement is confined to the rectum (proctitis) are not at increased risk.
2. *Primary sclerosing cholangitis (PSC).* Patients with UC have an increased risk of developing PSC, a chronic, progressive destructive disease of the cells that line the bile ducts. Patients with both PSC and chronic UC have an increased risk of developing dysplasia (altered appearance under the microscope of the cells lining the colon which is indicative of susceptibility to develop malignancy). The clinical characteristics of cancer in UC include:
   a. *Age of diagnosis.* The average age of diagnosis is 40 to 50 years, which is 10 to 20 years younger than cancer occurring in the general population.
   b. *Anatomic distribution.* Colorectal cancer occurs more evenly distributed throughout the colon compared to the general population in which 60% occurs in the sigmoid and rectum.
   c. *Survival.* When comparing diagnosis at equivalent pathologic stage, survival in both UC–associated cancer and in the general population is equivalent.

Genetic Mechanisms Underlying the Development of Cancer

Cancer in all its forms is essentially a disorder of gene regulation. In normal cells, cellular control mechanisms limit growth and division. The genes that play a major role in control of growth are called oncogenes and tumor suppressor genes. When cells escape from these controls, excessive growth and multiplication occur. Multiple abnormalities of those genes have been identified in the development of cancer from the normal epithelium (cells on the inner lining of the colon) to the malignant state.

Pathologic Features

Carcinoma complicating UC can assume a variety of appearances ranging from a flat, plaque-like format to a polypoid growth (protruding from the surface). Occasionally, malignancies can cause narrowing of the bowel wall (stricture formation).

Pathway of Development of Cancer in Ulcerative Colitis

It is important to understand that noncolitic cancers usually develop from an adenoma (commonly referred to as a polyp or adenomatous polyp), which is a benign tumor of the inner lining of the colon. Such benign tumors are dysplastic, a term that implies dysregulation of the architectural appearance of the cells when viewed under the microscope. It has been known for over 30 years that a similar but not identical process occurs in UC. Dysplasia occurring in UC (or CD) is often flat or plaque-like, but it similarly may be a precursor to the development of cancer. Dysplasia in IBD is thought to result from the repetitive cycle of inflammation and healing that occurs in the course of the illness.

Classification of Dysplasia

As pathologists have gained experience in recognizing dysplasia in the colonic specimens they have studied, a classification system has been developed that includes four possible diagnoses: negative (for dysplasia), indefinite, low grade, and high grade. Unfortunately, it does require considerable experience on the part of pathologists to reliably make the diagnosis of dysplasia.

Natural History of Dysplasia

While it can be conceptually convenient to expect that there may be an orderly progression from normal to low-grade to high-grade dysplasia to cancer (see below), the pace of evolution varies considerably from individual to individual. It must also be understood that there is no certainty that every patient with dysplasia will develop cancer although surveillance procedures to be discussed later make this presumption to provide for the safety of the individual patient.

Normal → low-grade dysplasia → high-grade dysplasia → cancer

Because of the somewhat subjective nature of pathologic interpretation, attempts have been made to develop more objective measures of cellular abnormality. One such technique involves the measurement of the amount of DNA in a population of colonic epithelial (lining) cells obtained by biopsy. Such measurements are quantified by instruments that measure the intensity of fluorescence in an individual cell. In general, areas of the colon that are dysplastic tend to have abnormalities of DNA content and are referred to as aneuploid. However, methodologic differences between laboratories and the somewhat specialized nature of this measurement have limited the widespread application of this technology.

Patient Management

The management possibilities for patients at increased risk for colorectal cancer include prophylactic proctocolectomy (removal of entire colon and rectum) or periodic surveillance (inspection of lining cells through a colonoscope with multiple biopsies of the cells by means of a forceps passed through one of the channels of the colonoscope). An onset of total UC in childhood or adolescence may convey a sufficiently great risk to warrant prophylactic proctocolectomy. At first glance, this may seem fairly radical but it would alleviate many years of endoscopic surveillance. On the other hand, the other issues that must be considered when making such a decision include the difficulties that may result from the presence of an ileostomy. However, newer techniques such as the ileal pouch–anal anastomosis may be well suited for young individuals. The decision to recommend a prophylactic proctocolectomy must be based on a detailed understanding of the individual patient. Intractability of symptoms, age, and psychological factors all must play a role in the ultimate decision. The patient and family must be educated about the objectives of long-term care so as to understand fully the different treatment alternatives.

Surveillance

The rationale for endoscopic surveillance in UC is based on several assumptions. These are that dysplasia is a consequence of long-standing colitis; that dysplasia is a reliable marker for cancer; and that surveillance detects cancer at an earlier stage than would be the case if one did not do surveillance, thereby improving survival. However, there have been no controlled trials of surveillance that have definitely proven that surveillance is effective in reducing death from cancer. However, it is the belief of many experienced gastroenterologists both in the United States and England that surveillance is clinically effective.

The aim of a surveillance program in chronic UC is not to detect early cancer but to detect early precancerous changes at a curable stage. In the early years of the illness, the extent of colonic involvement is determined by colonoscopic evaluation including biopsies. Subsequently, after 8 years of symptoms and the presence of extensive colitis (extending to at least the hepatic flexure), colonoscopies and biopsies are obtained annually. In those with left-sided colitis, it is probably reasonable to begin surveillance after 12 to 15 years of the disease. Multiple biopsies are obtained at 10 to 12 cm intervals through the entire colon and rectum.

It is essential to have the biopsy samples reviewed by a pathologist familiar with the interpretation of dysplasia. Communication between the gastroenterologist and pathologist is essential to minimize any misunderstandings about the significance of any endoscopic or pathologic findings.

Clinical Interpretation

Although controversy still exists about the value of endoscopic surveillance, many experienced clinicians use the following approach (2).

If the biopsies are classified as negative or indefinite, continued surveillance at 1-year intervals is advised. If low-grade or high-grade dysplasia is found, colectomy is indicated. In the past, some individuals have equivocated about the correct action in the presence of low-grade dysplasia preferring instead to perform follow-up colonoscopy in 3 to 6 months. If low-grade dysplasia was again found, then colectomy was advised. However, the difficulty inherent in this approach is that because the biopsies cover only a very small part of the surface area of the colon, it may be possible to miss the area of dysplastic involvement, thereby gaining a false sense of security.

Crohn's Disease

There appears to be an increased risk of colonic cancer in individuals with longstanding, extensive involvement of the colon. Although dysplasia is well recognized in the colon in CD, surveillance may be limited by the presence of stricture and fistulous disease. In patients with anorectal disease, prospective surveillance of the distal large bowel may be appropriate by utilizing the flexible sigmoidoscope to obtain the biopsies.

Summary

Cancer is a complication of chronic UC but is not as common as was once feared. Patient management for those at risk of cancer should be individualized. In the face of extensive, long-standing involvement of the colon by UC, management options include periodic surveillance or prophylactic proctocolectomy in the hope of preventing the development of colorectal cancer. Experience with surveillance in specialized centers that emphasize close collaboration between experienced gastroenterologists and pathologists suggests that this is safe.

REFERENCES

1. Levin B. Gastrointestinal neoplasia in inflammatory bowel disease. In: Kirsner JB, Shorter RG, eds. *Inflammatory bowel disease.* Baltimore: Williams & Wilkins, 1995;461–473.
2. Lennard-Jones JE. Prevention of cancer mortality in inflammatory bowel disease. In: Young GP, Rozen P, Levin B, eds. *Prevention and early detection of colorectal cancer.* Philadelphia: WB Saunders, 1996;218–238.

CHAPTER 6

INFLAMMATORY BOWEL DISEASE AND PREGNANCY

Lawrence J. Saubermann and Jacqueline L. Wolf

Most individuals with inflammatory bowel disease (IBD) develop it during their reproductive years. Therefore, issues pertaining to fertility, pregnancy, and the risk of inheritance of IBD become very important. Understanding how IBD affects the outcome of pregnancy and how pregnancy affects the IBD is essential information for the patient, spouse, and physician. Furthermore, nutrition, medication usage, diagnostic tests, and surgery may affect the outcome of a pregnancy in IBD patients. Despite all of these issues, the majority of individuals with IBD will have normal reproductive function and give birth to normal healthy full-term infants. The following discussion is designed to provide a better understanding of how IBD and its treatment impacts reproduction and pregnancy, and

Department of Gastroenterology, Brigham and Women's Hospital, and Harvard Medical School, Boston, Massachusetts 02115

how pregnancy impacts IBD. This information is provided as an overview and reference source, but not as a substitute for good medical care during pregnancy and continued interaction of the patient, the obstetrician, and the gastroenterologist.

FERTILITY

Fertility is not affected in women with IBD, except in rare instances. In men, sulfasalazine (Azulfidine, Pharmacia and Upjohn, Kalamazoo, MI) causes reversible changes in sperm that may lead to a temporary decrease in fertility. In contrast, sulfasalazine has no known effect on female fertility. The newer 5-aminosalicylic acid (5-ASA) compounds (Pentasa [Hoechst Marion Roussel, Kansas City, MO], Rowasa [Solvay, Marietta, GA], Asacol [Procter & Gamble Pharmaceuticals, Cincinnati, OH], Dipentum [Pharmacia and Upjohn, Kalamazoo, MI]) do not appear to affect the sperm or fertility. Hence, a man on sulfasalazine could be changed to one of these compounds if contemplating impregnation of his spouse. Decreases in female fertility that have been reported in the medical literature are either direct consequences of severe disease, malnutrition, or voluntary infrequency of intercourse. Intercourse frequency may be reduced because of fear of gas or stool passage during intercourse or the possibility of pain during intercourse.

EFFECT OF INFLAMMATORY BOWEL DISEASE ON PREGNANCY

There is general agreement among the specialists that in ulcerative colitis (UC), there is no significant effect of mild or inactive disease on pregnancy except for a 2 to 3 times increased risk of premature (before 37 weeks) birth (6% to 8%). This has been demonstrated in a few large reviews of pregnancies in women with colitis. However, when the activity is more severe, there is an increased risk to the fetus with higher incidences of spontaneous abortions above that in the general population.

Similarly, in Crohn's disease (CD), the degree of activity is associated with outcome. Approximately 85% to 90% of women with inactive or quiescent CD will have a normal pregnancy. Like UC, there is

TABLE 1. *Effect of inflammatory bowel disease on pregnancy*

- Sulfasalazine but not other 5-ASA medications cause reversible effects on sperm with a temporary decrease in fertility.
- Preterm (before 37 weeks) birth is increased in Crohn's disease and ulcerative colitis patients.
- In inactive disease, outcome of pregnancy is the same as in the healthy population.
- In active disease, there is a slightly increased risk of miscarriage and stillbirth.

an increased risk of premature birth (11% to 17%) although the risk is higher when active disease is present. Also, if the disease is active, there is an increased risk of spontaneous abortion and low birth weight. This appears to be irrespective of the site of intestinal involvement (large and/or small bowel). There is no contraindication to pregnancy when CD is inactive. In this case the outcome is expected to be the same as in a woman without IBD except for an increased risk of premature delivery. Although the overall effects of IBD on pregnancy are small, they appear to be associated with a more active disease state. Therefore, it would be advisable for a woman to consider becoming pregnant when her disease is inactive (Table 1).

EFFECTS OF PREGNANCY ON IBD

There is no increased rate of relapse in pregnant women with inactive UC compared to nonpregnant women. If a relapse occurs, then it generally occurs during the first two trimesters of pregnancy or following delivery. The rate of relapse for pregnant women with UC is approximately 34%. However, if someone has active UC at the time of pregnancy, then the activity generally continues without stopping during the course of their pregnancy, and 46% of women may notice a worsening of symptoms. Occasionally, the pregnancy may result in improvement in an individual's disease.

In CD, the rate of relapse for quiescent or inactive disease during pregnancy is approximately 27%. If relapse occurs, it happens most often during the first trimester or following delivery. During pregnancy 33% of women with active CD will notice a worsening of their symptoms, while approximately the same number will notice improvement.

TABLE 2. *Effect of pregnancy on inflammatory bowel disease*

- Pregnant women with inactive disease relapse at the same rate as nonpregnant women.
- Relapses, when they occur, generally occur in the first trimester and post partum, as well as in the second trimester for ulcerative colitis.
- Active disease at conception will remain active or worsen more than 65% of the time.

The risk of UC or CD flares in future pregnancies is unknown. Termination of a pregnancy does not appear to result in amelioration of IBD activity, and should only be considered for other reasons (Table 2).

MEDICATIONS

Most women want to avoid any medications during pregnancy and while nursing, but very often in patients with IBD it is necessary to treat the condition with some form of medication. Luckily, most of the medications used in IBD are safe in pregnancy and during breast-feeding (Table 3).

The *5-ASA compounds,* such as sulfasalazine (Azulfidine, Pharmacia and Upjohn, Kalamazoo, MI), mesalamine (Asacol, Pentasa, Rowasa), and olsalazine (Dipentum), are used to cause and maintain remission in IBD. Sulfasalazine has been in use for many decades and appears to be safe during pregnancy, as well as during nursing. Although there have been rare reports of congenital defects in women taking sulfasalazine, the incidence of defects is not increased over those in healthy women and did not prove to be due to the sulfasalazine. Ani-

TABLE 3. *Treatment of inflammatory bowel disease in pregnancy*

- Sulfasalazine, 5-aminosalicylic acid compounds, and corticosteroids appear to be safe for use in pregnancy.
- Loperamide can be used to control diarrhea.
- Azathioprine and 6-mercaptopurine may or may not be associated with a slight increase in birth defects or underweight babies.
- Cyclosporine A is associated with a 40% risk of premature birth.
- Do not use methotrexate.
- Do not use ciprofloxacin.

mal studies also show no effect of sulfasalazine on the fetus. Sulfasalazine interferes with folate activity in the body, but problems in nervous system development found in some women with folate deficiency are not increased in IBD patients. Folic acid supplementation should be used at all times when sulfasalazine is used and probably in all normal pregnancies. The amount of sulfasalazine transferred to the infant while nursing is small and appears to pose no risk. Newer preparations of 5-ASA compounds have not been tested to the same degree during pregnancy as sulfasalazine. Studies of 17 and 165 women with IBD who were undergoing treatment with oral mesalamine (Asacol) had successful pregnancies. One case report raised questions in regard to possible problems with the kidney in one infant but this may have been coincidental. Reversible watery diarrhea in a breast-feeding infant of a mother on Rowasa suppositories has also been described.

Corticosteroids remain the mainstay therapy for inducing remission in more severe forms of IBD. They have a long history of use in many other disease states as well. Thus their effects on pregnancy and in nursing mothers have been well evaluated. No congenital abnormalities are associated with steroid usage in women, and it appears to be safe in pregnancy. Women who are taking steroids appear to have an increased risk for premature deliveries and other fetal complications, but this may be due to their having an active disease that requires steroids. Although the steroids cross into the breast milk, they are not in concentrations great enough to affect the infant and are thus considered safe.

Azathioprine (Imuran, Glaxo Wellcome, Research Triangle Park, NC*) and 6-mercaptopurine (6-MP)* are immunosuppressive medications used in maintaining remissions and helping individuals lower or terminate their steroid usage. Information on their safety in pregnancy comes primarily from their safety record in organ transplant patients. Reviews of large numbers of cases show that about a 4% to 5% risk of congenital malformations are associated with these medications. This can be considered slightly above that in the normal population where it is 1% to 3%. There is no pattern to these malformations. There is, however, a significant increase in fetal growth retardation and prematurity in pregnant women on these immunosuppressives. Approximately one third of the pregnancies of individuals on azathioprine will result in infants who are small for their age.

Other risks to the fetus which are very rare include bone marrow suppression and immunosuppression in the newborn. These could cause anemia, increased risk of bleeding, or increased risk of infection. There appear to be no ill effects on fertility. Also, case reports of azathioprine and 6-MP usage during the time of conception up to the third trimester in women with IBD have shown no problems to the infants. As the medication can cross into breast milk, breast-feeding is not recommended until further information is obtained.

Cyclosporine A (Bristol-Myers Squibb, Princeton, NJ) is an immunosuppressive that affects the T-lymphocyte cells and is used in IBD primarily for short-term treatment of severe UC flares. At this time, only one case of cyclosporine A usage has been described in a pregnant woman with a UC flare at 29 weeks and the outcome was favorable. In other diseases, cyclosporine A usage has been associated with fetal growth retardation and prematurity in 40% of pregnancies. It does not appear to cause congenital malformations or fertility problems. Breast-feeding while on cyclosporine A is not recommended as the medication does cross into breast milk and the effects are not known.

Methotrexate (Roxane, Columbus, OH) an immunosuppressive agent that is used to induce and maintain a remission in individuals with IBD, should not be used in pregnancy. One of its uses in high doses is to induce abortions during the first trimester. Reports of pregnancies in which it was used to treat non-IBD disease demonstrate that methotrexate is clearly associated with an increased, dose-related, risk of congenital malformations during the 6- to 8-week period after conception. Growth retardation is found in approximately 40% of infants and bone marrow toxicity has been reported. Reversible fertility problems have occurred in both men and women taking the medication. The mother should not breast-feed while taking methotrexate because the breast milk can contain the medication, although the amount in breast milk is small compared to that in the mother's blood. Pregnancy should be delayed until several months after the drug is stopped.

Metronidazole (Flagyl, Searle, Chicago, IL) is an antibiotic used to treat some cases of IBD. Its effect on pregnant individuals with IBD is not well known. The data from comprehensive reviews of women who became pregnant while on the medication suggest that it is safe. However, given the results from studies in animals, unless absolutely necessary, its use should be restricted to the third trimester. It is expressed in breast milk, and it is currently recommended that women on this medication not breast-feed.

Ciprofloxacin (Cipro) (Bayer Corporation, West Haven, CT) is an antibiotic used to treat selective cases of IBD. In some puppies, it has been shown to affect developing cartilage, resulting in chronic arthritis. In a group of women with urinary tract infections who received the medication during the first trimester, no malformations occurred, but there was an increase in the cesarean rate. Because its effects on the human fetus are not known, it is recommended that pregnant women avoid the use of ciprofloxacin during pregnancy and while breast-feeding.

Other agents used in IBD include antidiarrheals, bulk fiber, and cholestyramine. *Loperamide (Imodium,* McNeil Consumer, Fort Washington, PA) appears safe with no reported ill effects on pregnancy, whereas *diphenoxylate with atropine (Lomotil,* Searle and Co., Chicago, IL) has been reported to cause impaired fertility and decreased maternal weight gain. Therefore, loperamide appears to be the preferred antidiarrheal during pregnancy when needed for IBD and is considered safe for breast-feeding. *Kaopectin (Kaopectate,* Pharmacia and Upjohn, Kalamazoo, MI) and *bulk fiber (Metamucil,* Procter and Gamble, Cincinnati, OH) are also considered safe in pregnancy and during breast-feeding. *Cholestyramine* is not taken up by the body but does affect the absorption of vitamins; therefore, vitamin supplementation should be given in conjunction with cholestyramine. There does not appear to be any ill effects from the medication on pregnancy or while nursing.

NURSING

Nursing is considered safe for women with IBD and is recommended for the development of the infant. The only issue pertaining to nursing with IBD is the risk of the mother's medications crossing into the breast milk and affecting the infant. As noted above, most medications are safe, but certain medications should not be used in the nursing mother. If the medication is absolutely required, then other supplemental nutrition may be necessary.

NUTRITION

Nutrition is fundamental to the growth and development of the fetus during pregnancy. A well-balanced diet with adequate calcium, iron, and vitamins is essential. This aspect of maternal care can sometimes be difficult to manage during an acute flare of IBD. Occasionally, bowel rest may be required to improve symptoms or allow healing of fistulas or strictures. In pregnant women with active CD, an elemental diet (i.e., one in which the food has already been broken down enough to allow easy absorption) can provide adequate nutrition and may induce remission. This method of feeding represents a possible alternative to the more standard total parenteral nutrition (TPN) whereby the nutrition is supplied directly into the bloodstream through a needle and catheter.

SURGERY

Whenever possible, surgery should be avoided during pregnancy. However, if the disease is severe and not responding to drug therapy, then it may be more dangerous to the individual's health not to operate. Emergency surgery is associated with an increased risk of postoperative spontaneous abortions.

In women with perineal or anal disease, cesarean section should not be done routinely with the hope of avoiding rectal complications following a vaginal delivery. Although patients can develop problems at an episiotomy site, vaginal deliveries have been done without difficulty. When an episiotomy is done, it is important that the obstetrician do it away from any present fistula or fissure. It is unclear as to the degree of anal and perineal involvement that would benefit from cesarean versus vaginal deliveries.

Women with an ileal pouch–anal anastomosis do well during and after pregnancy. There is only a slight increase in daytime and nighttime stools which can persist up to 3 months after delivery. The type of delivery, whether vaginal or cesarean, appears to have no effect on stool continence or frequency post delivery in these women. Following ileostomy construction, most physicians suggest that pregnancy be delayed for about a year to allow the body time to heal and adapt. There is a slight increased risk of ileostomy prolapse and obstruction and an increase in stool output in pregnant women with ileostomies.

DIAGNOSTIC TESTS

Common endoscopic procedures such as colonoscopy (examination of the large intestine), flexible sigmoidoscopy (examination of the last part of the large intestine), and upper intestinal endoscopy (EGD) are well tolerated during the pregnant state and appear to be safe. Examination of the pancreatic and bile duct with a scope (endoscopic retrograde cholangiopancreatography, ERCP), has also been performed during pregnancy without any higher complication rate than in the non-pregnant state. The fetal heart rate should be measured before and after the procedure. Continuous monitoring of the fetal heart is optional and may be considered. The pregnant woman receiving sedation should have her vital signs and oxygen level monitored during the procedure as well. The medications used are generally safe for the short duration of the procedure, although meperidine (Demerol, Sanofi Winthrop, New York, NY) or fentanyl may be safer than diazepam (Valium, Roche Products, Manati, Puerto Rico) or midazolam (Versed, Roche Laboratories, Nutley, NJ). Concerns should be addressed with the physician performing the procedure.

Ultrasonography is used frequently in obstetric care to monitor development of the fetus and is felt to be safe to use during pregnancy.

Magnetic resonance imaging (MRI) is a new method for examining internal body structures. Few data are available in pregnancy, but it is probably safe and can be used to image the abdomen if necessary for an IBD-associated problem.

Computed axial tomography (CAT) scan and x-rays result in radiation exposure to the fetus and thus are not routinely used. Occasionally, it becomes necessary to use these tests for diagnosis. When used, x-ray exposure should be limited to the minimum number of views possible.

HEREDITY

There are clear indications that genetic factors play a role in IBD. No specific gene has been identified in IBD, though research into many possibilities continues. There have been multiple reports showing that a family history of IBD is a strong predictor of subsequent disease, with an increased incidence in identical twins. In recent studies of families, the age of onset as well as the location of the disease appear to run in families. If one parent has IBD, there is approximately an 8% to 10% chance of inheriting the disease, and, according to one study, if two parents have IBD the likelihood of inheriting the disease increases to up to 36%. The risk of inheriting the disease is less in UC than in CD and may be less in the non-Jewish than the Jewish population. At this time, there is no definite way to predict who will or will not develop IBD, and decisions with regard to conception will need to be individually addressed.

SUMMARY

In most women with IBD, pregnancy is safe and the delivery of a healthy baby is not affected by the disease. Even though the effects of IBD on reproduction and pregnancy are for the most part minimal, certain considerations need to be addressed to improve outcome. Pregnancies certainly do better if the individual is in an inactive or quiescent disease state. Nutrition should be maintained in association with frequent and close supervision of the gastroenterologist and obstetrician. Also, medications should be reviewed and either adjusted or changed if required to avoid complications. Finally, though the risk of inheritance of IBD in the offspring can occur, there is no way to currently predict whether or not any given child will develop the disease.

ACKNOWLEDGMENT

The authors thank Ms. Liles Smith for her expert assistance in preparing the manuscript.

SUGGESTED READINGS

Alstead EM, Ritchie JK, Lennard-Jones JE, Farthing MJ, Clark ML. Safety of azathioprine in pregnancy in inflammatory bowel disease. *Gastroenterology* 1990; 99:443–446.

Baird DD, Narendranathan M, Sandler RS. Increased risk of preterm birth for women with inflammatory bowel disease. *Gastroenterology* 1990;99:987–994.

Bermas BL, Hill JA. Effects of immunosuppressive drugs during pregnancy. *Arthritis Rheum* 1995;38:1722–1732.

Brandt LJ, Estabrook SG, Reinus JF. Results of a survey to evaluate whether vaginal delivery and episiotomy lead to perineal involvement in women with Crohn's disease. *Am J Gastroenterol* 1995;90:1918–1922.

Connell WR. Safety of drug therapy for inflammatory bowel disease in pregnant and nursing women. *Inflam bowel dis* 1996;2:33–47.

Diav-Citrin O, Park YH, Veerasuntharam G, et al. The safety of mesalamine in human pregnancy: a prospective controlled cohort study. *Gastroenerology* 1998; 114:23–28.

Juhasz ES, Fozard B, Dozois RR, Ilstrup DM, Nelson H. Ileal pouch-anal anastomosis function following childbirth: an extended evaluation. *Dis Colon Rectum* 1995;38:159–165.

Lewis JH, Weingold AB. The use of gastrointestinal drugs during pregnancy and lactation. *Am J Gastroenterol* 1985;80:912–923.

Mayberry JF, Weterman IT. European survey of fertility and pregnancy in women with Crohn's disease: a case control study by European Collaborative Group. *Gut* 1986;27:821–825.

Metcalf AM, Dozois RR, Kelly KA. Sexual function in women after proctocolectomy. *Ann Surg* 1986;204:624–627.

Miller JP. Inflammatory bowel disease in pregnancy: a review. *J R Soc Med* 1986;79:221–225.

Ostensen M. Treatment with immunosuppressive and disease modifying drugs during pregnancy and lactation. *Am J Reprod Immunol* 1992;28:148–152.

Sjogren B, Poppen B. Sexual life in women after colectomy-proctomucosectomy with S-pouch. *Acta Obstet Gynecol Scand* 1995;74:51–55.

Teahon K, Pearson M, Levi AJ, Bjarnason I. Elemental diet in the management of Crohn's disease during pregnancy. *Gut* 1991;32:1079–1081.

Woolfson K, Cohen Z, McLeod RS. Crohn's disease and pregnancy. *Dis Colon Rectum* 1990; 33:869–873.

Yang H, McElree C, Roth MP, Shanahan F, Targan SR, Rotter JI. Familial empiric risks for inflammatory bowel disease: differences between Jews and non-Jews. *Gut* 1993;34:517–524.

CHAPTER 7

INFLAMMATORY BOWEL DISEASE IN CHILDREN AND ADOLESCENTS

*Susan N. Peck and
*¶David A. Piccoli

Inflammatory bowel disease (IBD) is the most common chronic gastrointestinal illness in children and adolescents. About one third of all patients with Crohn's disease (CD) and ulcerative colitis (UC) have the onset of their illness before adulthood. The diseases may occur as early as the first few years of life, but the peak age is in adolescence. While there are many similarities in the manifestations of the disease and its therapy in children compared to adults, there are also many important differences. These add to the complexity and

Division of Gastroenterology and Nutrition, The Children's Hospital of Philadelphia, and ¶Department of Pediatrics, University of Pennsylvania School of Medicine, Philadelphia, Pennsylvania 19104

challenge of caring for children with IBD. Pediatric gastroenterologists have developed an approach to IBD that focuses on the growing child and the family.

The growth and development that must occur in late childhood and early adolescence is an important concern. Growth requires significant nutrients that may be severely depleted in a patient with a poor appetite. Nutrients may also be lost through an inflamed intestinal tract. Additionally, medications such as prednisone further inhibit normal growth. The poor growth seen in so many children has its own effect on the general health and psychological well-being of a young patient and adds to the challenges posed by the chronic illness itself. Medical therapies developed to treat IBD have only been tested in adults. While these medications are prescribed carefully for young patients, the exact dosages have not been established for children. Each aspect of a child's care must take into consideration the patient's stage of growth and development. The long-term implications of care must be considered, as children with CD and UC may have dealt with decades of disease by the time they become young adults. This duration of disease forces patients to deal with the consequences and risks of long-term illness at a relatively young age. A team approach is utilized in most centers in an effort to provide families with the education and support needed for living with a chronic disease.

PRESENTATION OF CROHN'S DISEASE AND ULCERATIVE COLITIS IN CHILDREN AND ADOLESCENTS

CD and UC have a wide range of symptoms in children and adolescents, and a delay in diagnosis is common, as many of the symptoms do not at first suggest IBD. In children, there are many other types of inflammatory bowel diseases that are not CD or UC. These causes must be considered, as most of them are curable with therapy. Infections of the bowel causing inflammation are common at all ages and are much more common than IBD in young children. Stool cultures and collections can identify most organisms and guide specific therapy. *Salmonella, Shigella,* invasive *E. coli,* and *Clostridium difficile* are a few of the bacterial infections that can mimic signs of

IBD in children. Tuberculosis of the intestines and the parasitic infection amebiasis can also look like IBD. Allergies to protein in formula can cause colitis in infants. In sick infants, a particularly aggressive form of ileitis and colitis called necrotizing enterocolitis (NEC) can occur. Infants with severe abnormalities of the immune system may also have colitis. In older children and adolescents, some patients may have symptoms that suggest endocrine, kidney, or infectious diseases.

Almost all children and adolescents with UC have diarrhea and rectal bleeding at the time of diagnosis. Most also have abdominal pain. One third have weight loss, and 10% have growth failure. Rarely, a patient will have joint inflammation (arthritis or joint pain) or fevers before any bowel symptoms occur. Patients with CD may have symptoms similar to those of UC, but rectal bleeding is much less common. The most common symptoms of pediatric CD are abdominal pain and fever. Diarrhea is less common, and the absence of diarrhea can lead to a delay in diagnosis. Malnutrition and growth retardation are much more common in CD than UC and occur in over one third of patients. Joint disease is also more common in patients with CD. Perianal disease occurs in one fourth of patients with Crohn's but is extremely uncommon in children with UC. CD is diagnosed in some children when they develop pain that appears to be due to appendicitis.

More commonly, the onset of CD is gradual, and there is often a long delay between the first symptoms and the eventual diagnosis. Often the symptoms are subtle and may mimic other diseases. Abdominal pain is a common problem in healthy children, and specific features of CD may be absent. Growth retardation may not be noticed unless a patient's heights and weights are plotted on a growth curve. Although infant growth curves are routinely used, the growth rates of older school age patients are plotted less commonly by physicians or schools. Parents may note, however, that a child's shoe, belt, or pant size has not changed for a significant period of time. Some patients with malnutrition have lost weight, but more commonly they have simply failed to gain weight at the expected rate for their age. In either situation, this lack of appropriate weight gain can result in failure to grow appropriately in height. This lack of height gain can result in permanent short stature if it is not successfully treated. Growth failure also signifies that a patient has significant deficiencies of minerals and nutrients. Growth failure is commonly associated with a delay in sexual maturation and a late onset of puberty. At times the severe delay in growth and puberty will result in an evaluation for endocrine disease if no bowel symptoms are present to suggest IBD. Adolescents with unexplained weight loss and poor intake may be mistakenly thought to have anorexia nervosa. The combination of fevers, weight loss, and a mass in the abdomen can be mistaken for cancer. Occasionally, a patient will only have unexplained fevers at the onset of IBD.

DIAGNOSTIC STUDIES FOR CROHN'S DISEASE AND ULCERATIVE COLITIS

The diagnostic evaluation of IBD in children relies on the same tests used in adults. Radiographic studies can be performed by a specialized radiologist with an expertise in pediatrics. Endoscopy is necessary for diagnosis, even in infants. This can be performed safely, with minimal psychological and physical trauma. Special endoscopes have been developed for smaller patients, and these tests can now be performed in children of all ages. Adequate sedation is essential for the successful completion of an endoscopic study, and preparation of the patient in advance by experienced personnel is helpful. The use of intravenous sedation in pediatric facilities is well standardized and safe. At times, general anesthesia may be necessary. Children generally tolerate sedation or anesthesia well, and many have little memory of the procedure. Most procedures are performed in an outpatient setting, unless the severity of the patient's illness necessitates hospitalization.

DIAGNOSTIC CRITERIA FOR CROHN'S DISEASE, ULCERATIVE COLITIS, AND INDETERMINATE COLITIS

The criteria for the diagnosis of pediatric CD and UC are the same as those used for adults. Colitis is documented by barium enema or, more commonly, by endoscopy and biopsies of the colon. Intestinal inflammation in the small intestine, or ileitis, is identified by upper GI series with a small bowel follow-through, or when the endoscopist is able to obtain biopsies from the terminal ileum at colonoscopy. Patients with small bowel disease or intermittent areas of inflammation (skip areas) have CD, as do patients with granulomas seen on biopsy of the bowel. Patients with colitis that extends upward from the rectum without skip areas and without ileitis have a pattern consistent with UC.

A small number of young patients have a type of colitis that cannot be definitively classified as Crohn's colitis or UC. To reflect this uncertainty, these patients are diagnosed with indeterminate colitis. Further testing, sometimes years after diagnosis, may identify the specific diagnosis. In the future, specific laboratory or genetic testing may help to differentiate the diseases. Although the medical therapy is similar for pediatric CD and UC, there are dramatic differences in the surgical therapy. Extra care must be taken in patients for whom a final diagnosis has not been established.

MEDICAL THERAPY

Medications are an integral part of the therapy for IBD, and several types of medications may be necessary to control the disease. The medical therapy for IBD in children and adolescents is similar to the approach in adults. There are, however, many special considerations. Toddlers may require therapy in the first few years of life, but the safety and effectiveness of most IBD medications have not been tested in young children. Although it appears that medications are effective and generally safe, large studies of the effects and the side effects of many medications in pediatric patients have not been performed.

Some medications, however, have significantly different side effects in the pediatric population. Prednisone is the most important example. Prednisone causes a significant slowing of linear (height) growth, even when a patient's nutritional status is adequate. In most patients with IBD the negative effects of prednisone on height are added to the negative effects of malnutrition. Long-term administration of prednisone can result in significant delays in height gain. In adults maximal height has already been attained, so that the growth complication is not an issue. The other bone complications of prednisone, particularly osteoporosis or softening of the bones, is similar in children and adults. Because so much effort is placed on attaining normal growth, the side effects of chronic prednisone use may be intolerable for many patients. As a result, many pediatric medication strategies are designed to eliminate the reliance on prednisone. These approaches include use of immunomodulatory agents, nutritional therapy, or surgical resection. Use of the immunomodulatory agents 6-mercaptopurine and azathioprine will allow the majority of young patients to markedly decrease or eliminate the need for prednisone therapy. Nasogastric alimentation can markedly improve growth and diminish the need for prednisone in some patients. Several studies have shown that surgical resection in prepubertal patients with favorable disease anatomy will result in a growth spurt and a decrease in prednisone dependency. The timing of these strategies is critically important. If a patient has passed the peak growth potential, then "steroid-sparing" strategies will be ineffective.

Most medications developed to treat IBD are designed to be given to adults. While these medications can be safely prescribed for children, there are a number of problems that may be encountered. Exact dosages for children have not been established for many of the medications. Timed release preparations are designed to be released in a much longer and generally slower adult intestine.

An additional problem may occur because IBD medications may not be "kid-friendly." The commercial preparations are difficult or impossible for young children to swallow. Many are available only in pill or capsule, and some are very large. Liquid preparations, when available, may have a particularly unpleasant taste that requires camouflage. The most common medications used to treat IBD in children are the 5-aminosalicylates (5-ASA) (sulfasalazine, olsalazine, and mesalamine). None of the 5-ASA medications are commercially available as liquids, and only sulfasalazine (Azulfidine) may be made into a suspension by a willing and knowledgeable pharmacist. Pentasa (Hoechst Marion Rouseel, Kansas City, MO) (mesalamine) capsules may be opened and mixed in food such as applesauce or ice cream, but Asacol (Procter and Gamble, Cincinnati, OH) (mesalamine) should be taken whole. It is not unusual to see the casing from an Asacol tablet or the beads from Pentasa in a child's stool.

The corticosteroids are powerful medications that have significant positive and negative effects on patients. Both prednisone and prednisolone have a bitter aftertaste. Prednisolone is available in a liquid suspension. However, the concentration of the suspension and the taste are obstacles for many children. A child who requires 30 mg of liquid prednisolone each day would require 2 tablespoons (1 oz) of medication each day. An alternative would be to give the child 2 tablets (one 20-mg tablet and one 10-mg tablet) crushed and mixed in a small amount of ice cream or applesauce, minimizing the amount and taste of the medication.

Enemas are helpful in treating IBD, but most children dislike having medicine inserted into the rectum. Medication enemas are more likely to be successful if done gently and in a supportive environment with good technique. The child should lie left side down, and it may be helpful to have him or her cuddle a toy or stuffed animal. Lubricate the suppository or enema tip with a water-soluble lubricant. Before inserting, ask the child to bear down as if having a bowel movement. This opens the anal sphincter and helps the child to relax. While the child bears down, give the medication at a steady, moderate pace. Encourage the child to take deep breaths if there is any discomfort. Older children and adolescents may prefer to administer rectal medications themselves and should be encouraged to do so. However, parents must be sure that they are actually taking the medication and not throwing it away. Both mesalamine (Rowasa) (Solvay, Marietta, GA) and hydrocortisone (steroids) are available in rectal preparations (enema and suppository).

It is difficult for adults and children alike to remember to take medicine at the appropriate times. Associating medicines with mealtimes or other routines may be helpful. Medications dosed 4 times a day should be taken with breakfast, lunch, dinner, and at bedtime. Three-times-a-day doses are taken with breakfast, after school, and at bedtime, and twice-daily doses at breakfast and dinner, or breakfast and bedtime. As children enter adolescence, medication compliance may become an issue. Peer pressure and the desire to be like everyone else impacts on decision making. Parents begin to expect children to take responsibility for their care, whereas the child may have little interest in assuming the responsibility or acknowledging that he or she has a chronic illness. It is during this phase of life that children stop their medications, usually without parental permission or knowledge. It is not uncommon to find medications hidden or wasted. Lifestyle also impacts on compliance. For the active adolescent, taking a medication 2 or 3 times a day is much easier than 4 times, and medication schedules should be adjusted accordingly. Children and adolescents need reminders, such as watches with alarms set for the after-school dose, marked calendars for alternate day steroids, or pill boxes with a week's supply of medications organized by day.

ROLE OF NUTRITION IN THE CARE OF PATIENTS WITH IBD

Proper nutrition is important for the care of any patient with IBD. Pediatric patients have special requirements that increase the need for calories and vitamins. The challenge is particularly difficult in CD where one third of young patients will have growth failure and two thirds will have deficiencies in minerals or vitamins. Inadequate nutrition is due to a combination of factors. Many patients lose calories and nutrients due to chronic diarrhea. Certain nutrients and vitamins (such as vitamin B_{12}) are absorbed primarily in one specific site in the intestine, and if this area is inflamed or removed by surgery, deficiencies will occur. The most important cause of malnutrition in pediatric CD is inadequate intake. This is due to poor appetite and to the symptoms that occur following eating in some patients. In order to document intake, families may complete a 3-day food diary, which is analyzed by computer to determine the adequacy of the patient's diet. Based on this information, specific counseling can be provided by a nutritionist to construct an adequate diet and correct deficiencies. The most important patient need is for total calories, or energy intake. These calories are the fuel for maintenance and growth. A patient with IBD needs energy for resting metabolism, exercise and activity, replacement of ongoing losses, correction of deficits, and growth. The basal metabolism requirements can be calculated from a patient's weight and age, or can be measured by a simple test called a resting energy expenditure (REE). The energy required for activity depends largely on a patient's lifestyle and can vary widely. Young athletes with IBD may require thousands of extra calories per day. Diarrhea may result in substantial losses of calories, nutrients, and protein. Patients with small intestinal CD may have protein-losing enteropathy, a condition in which high levels of protein are lost in the stool. Iron and minerals are commonly depleted in patients with chronic diarrhea. The diet must be specifically modified if these problems are present.

At diagnosis, many young patients have fallen off their growth curves. This growth failure is one of the major complications of CD in the pediatric population. Growth failure indicates that nutrient and energy depletion has occurred to such a degree that weight and height increases have slowed below the child's potential. This is a serious deficiency that must be corrected. Finally, unlike adults, children and adolescents require energy for growth. These energy needs continue until linear growth is completed, which in many patients is in the late teens. The energy needs of young patients are typically higher than for adults, and these needs can be accurately calculated. If a dietary analysis indicates that a patient is not taking adequate calories for catch-up growth, dietary counseling and nutritional supplements are recommended. Parents can construct a well-balanced diet with sufficient quantities of calories and protein to meet a child's increased needs. An extra meal at bedtime is a valuable addition. Vitamin supplementation is essential in patients with poor intake or significant losses. Nutritional supplements ("power shakes") provide extra calories and protein, and should be given in place of other fluids. The quality and taste of supplements has improved dramatically, but many young patients will not take the recommended quantities. Although nutrition is critically important, it is essential that mealtime not be a battle between well-meaning parents and a resistant child. Counseling and motivational therapy can help parents develop strategies to deal with the problem, but in many children supplements will not be effective because the child ultimately will not drink them.

As a result, other strategies are commonly employed in young adolescents with IBD. The most important of these is nasogastric tube feeding, or NG feeding. Overnight nasogastric tube feeding has been shown to be an effective therapy to provide catch-up growth and reverse growth failure. This is accomplished by infusing a high-calorie formula via a tube placed through the nose and into the stomach. The formula is pumped in overnight while the child is sleeping.

The type of formula, the hourly rate, and the length of the feedings will be determined by the health care team to meet the patient's nutritional and therapeutic goals. Nasogastric tube feeding sounds extreme but it is usually very successful. No parent looks forward to this intervention, and many doubt that they and their child can even do it. Education is essential if this approach is to work. The importance of nutrition must be stressed at all educational sessions. Patients should see their own growth curves and have a clear understanding of the goals of this therapy. Patients who understand the need for extra calories are more motivated to try tube feeding if they have tried and failed to take supplements. It is very helpful to have a veteran adolescent meet a patient considering this therapy. Support systems need to be in place for the parents and for their children. The keys to success are excellent teaching and an easy first demonstration. Parents and, in most cases, the adolescents themselves must learn to pass the tube into the stomach. In the presence of experienced and supportive nurses or physicians, this initial session can go smoothly and lead to long-term success. The feeding tubes are soft, small, very flexible silicone tubes that are about the size of a coffee stirrer. The nose and the back of the throat may be numbed before placement to decrease gagging and discomfort. The family is taught to measure the tube for correct placement. Passage of the tube is then demonstrated on a willing volunteer or a mannequin. Once comfortable with the basics, the child or parent passes the tube, demonstrating the ability to follow the steps and to confirm placement. The family is also instructed in the use of an enteral infusion pump. The actual brand of tube and enteral infusion pump varies with institutional and home care agencies. Home health care agencies provide supportive services for individuals on nasogastric feedings at home. Before starting NG therapy, it is essential to determine that insurance coverage is provided for this type of therapy. Some insurance plans will cover the cost of pumps and tubing, but not formula, which can be prohibitively expensive for some families.

After the first few days at home, even young patients adapt to the nightly passing of the tube and infusion of the formula. The great benefit of nasogastric alimentation, or feeding, is that it is possible to deliver very large quantities of formula regardless of taste while a young patient sleeps. There are two basic strategies for nasogastric alimentation. In the first, the formula is a supplement, or boost, to add to the child's daily intake. One or two thousand calories can be delivered overnight. Generally, this is enough to provide for excellent catch-up growth, increased energy levels, and correction of deficits. Many adolescents will administer this nasogastric supplementation for years, particularly around the time of the pubertal growth spurt. A second strategy is to use the NG tube to deliver all of the patient's nutrition. Some studies have suggested that this approach is as effective as medical therapy for active CD, with fewer risks. Generally, an elemental formula is used as the only protein intake. These formulas are not as palatable as standard supplements, and thus rarely will a patient take these very large quantities of supplements orally. Patients receiving this therapy may choose to leave the tube in place during the day, but patients receiving only supplemental feedings insert the tube at night and remove it in the morning. Although tube feeding is both expensive and relatively difficult, a large number of adolescents choose and remain with this regimen because of its dramatic success.

PSYCHOSOCIAL SUPPORT IN INFLAMMATORY BOWEL DISEASE

While there is no evidence that psychological factors such as stress or nerves play a role in the development of IBD, for many years IBD was believed to be a psychosomatic illness. That myth continues today. Well-intentioned family members and friends may comment on the nervous tendency of a child. Health care professionals may remark that they have an IBD personality. Living with a chronic illness such as CD or UC affects not only the child but the entire family. Rather than stress causing the disease, the disease causes stress. Recognizing the psychological impact of chronic illness is an important part of the management of IBD.

A team approach is useful for the management of pediatric IBD. The team often includes physicians, advanced practice nurses, procedure nurses, social workers, psychologists, and nutritionists. Each member offers a specific area of expertise for IBD. Recognizing that each patient is an individual, the involvement of some members of the team will vary depending on the needs of the child and family. It is important to involve the family and the community in supporting the child diagnosed with IBD.

Education is necessary to understand the implications of living with IBD. Children need basic knowledge regarding the disease process, the concepts of flares and remissions, the diagnostic process, and the therapeutic modalities. It is important for them to feel supported by their family and friends. They must be included in some of the decision making regarding their health care and they must feel part of the team. The age and developmental level of the child will dictate how and what he or she should hear and learn. There are many ways to learn about IBD. Videotapes provide a non-threatening forum for all age groups. Pamphlets detailing the diagnosis, and the medical, surgical, and nutritional options are available through the Crohn's and Colitis Foundation of America (CCFA). Education seminars sponsored by the CCFA offer families an opportunity to meet with experts. Children are provided the opportunity to learn about IBD through games and group activities.

SCHOOL ISSUES

School is an integral part of a child's life. Many aspects of IBD impact on how children are viewed by their friends, classmates, and teachers. Teachers have a profound influence over these interactions and should be aware of the child's medical condition. Teacher involvement may help avoid difficult and embarrassing situations. Children with IBD may appear younger and be smaller than their classmates. Medications may also result in changes in appearance. Prednisone, for example, may cause weight gain, a puffy appearance to the face, and acne. An informed teacher is able to intervene and support the child when classmates question or tease.

Attacks of pain and an urgent need to use the bathroom may occur suddenly and without warning. Many schools now lock the bathroom between classes and some have eliminated doors on the bathroom stalls for security reasons. Parents should investigate their child's school situation to help the school develop a plan to provide bathroom access at the nurse's office, which will often reduce the student's anxiety. A physician's note to the school stating the child's diagnosis will allow restroom privileges to be arranged in a way that eliminates calling attention to the child. A change of clothes can help considerably in unfortunate situations.

Children often need to take medications during school hours. Schools generally require written guidelines for medication administration. It is important for the school nurse to be aware of the child's medications and possible side effects. Medication administration should be arranged so that minimal attention is drawn to the child.

Participation in physical education classes should be encouraged. For some children with IBD, intense physical activity may aggravate their symptoms, but moderate activity is beneficial for all patients. Malnutrition and the manifestations of disease may limit a student's ability to perform, and school programs should be encouraged to make special considerations for ill patients. A modified gym program may be advisable, and in some cases a patient should be excused from participation. Children who have required prolonged steroid therapy may be at risk for fractures. Consultation with your physician is advisable prior to participation in contact sports such as football, basketball, or soccer.

Not all children with IBD appear small or ill, but they may be experiencing symptoms of their disease. Because they do not seem sick, it is easy for people to misjudge the extent of their illness. The goal of medical therapy is to keep the child as functional as possible, and school should be viewed as their career. Parents and children should be committed to their regular attendance at school. However, absences will occur due to flares of the disease and hospitalizations. Every effort should be made to help the child maintain his or her school work. Many school systems have child study teams that provide homebound tutoring without requiring a prolonged absence from school. When prolonged absences do occur, children appreciate hearing from their classmates and feeling that they are a part of the class. This will help to ease the transition back to the classroom after a long illness. Teachers should be encouraged to notify families of subtle changes in the child's performance or a change in behavior, such as needing to be excused from class frequently. Communication between the school and the health care team may also be helpful. The health care team should provide the school with written material regarding IBD to remove the myths and stigmas associated with CD and UC. When older students are away at boarding school or college, medical information should be transmitted to the school and a physician's visit should be arranged prior to the start of the school year.

LONG-TERM ISSUES

Patients with the onset of IBD in childhood face many obstacles. Their early childhood may be affected by the disease and its medical therapy. In addition to the normal stresses of growing up, they must face the challenges of chronic illness. The social challenges of adolescence can be magnified by the symptoms and complications of IBD. Before adulthood these patients may have to deal with the issues of cancer surveillance or elective surgery. If surgery is required in CD, every effort must be undertaken to decrease the risk of postoperative recurrence of the disease.

Families must anticipate future needs, such as medical and life insurance. Many centers have disease management programs that promote health and quality of life within the context of a chronic illness.

SUGGESTED READING

Benirschke R. *Alive and kicking*. San Diego: Firefly Press, 1996.
Benkov K, Winter H. *Managing your child's Crohn's disease or ulcerative colitis*. New York: CCFA/Mastermedia Ltd., 1996.

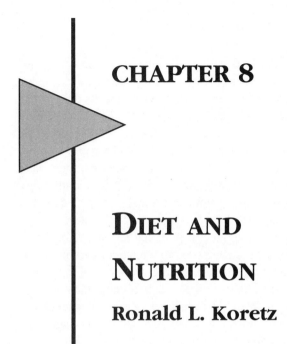

CHAPTER 8

DIET AND

NUTRITION

Ronald L. Koretz

"Some people have a foolish way of not minding, or pretending not to mind, what they eat. For my part, I mind my belly very studiously, and very carefully; for I look upon it, that he who does not mind his belly will hardly mind anything else."—Samuel Johnson

This chapter will deal with diet and nutrition as those topics apply to inflammatory bowel disease (IBD). We will first consider normal nutrition, so the subsequent terminology and concepts will be familiar. We will then look at two aspects of nutrition and IBD: (a) how IBD interferes with normal nutrition and (b) potential therapeutic interventions relating to the diet.

NORMAL NUTRITION

Nutrients

The diet is composed of sources of energy, protein, vitamins, and minerals. Although specific Recommended Daily Allowances (RDAs)

Department of Internal Medicine, Olive View-UCLA Medical Center, Sylmar,
California 91342; and UCLA School of Medicine, Los Angeles, California 90024

have been published, it is true that all people who consume a "normal" diet get enough of the various nutrients that they require.

Energy is the fuel that allows the body to carry out its daily activities. It is taken in as carbohydrate or as fat. If one absorbs more energy than the body needs, the extra is stored as fat; even if the energy is initially eaten as carbohydrate, the body converts it to fat. On the other hand, if one burns more than one absorbs, the excess need is obtained by tapping the fat reserves (the principle of dieting).

Fat contains more energy per gram (9 calories) than does carbohydrate (4 calories). Fats are also more complicated molecules. Fat usually is found in the form of triglycerides, which are three fatty acids linked together. A fatty acid is composed of a chain of carbon atoms; depending on how many such atoms there are, we speak of long chain (more than 12), medium-chain (4 to 12), or short chain fatty acids (2 or 3). Furthermore, the links in these chains may vary; biochemically, we talk about saturated and unsaturated bonds, but one can think about these as wires holding the carbon atoms together. A saturated bond would consist of one wire, whereas an unsaturated bond would be analogous to two wires tying the atoms together.

Fat can also be found as cholesterol. In this case, the carbon atoms are arranged in a series of interlocking circles (rather than as chains). Cholesterol-related molecules have different properties and metabolic fates than do the triglycerides. For instance, cholesterol is not a major source of energy, but these molecules are metabolized into certain hormones and bile acids.

Carbohydrates are substances that contain one or more sugar molecules (glucose, galactose, or fructose). When there is only a single molecule, we speak of "monosaccharides" (or each respective sugar name). Disaccharides consist of two of these molecules bound together; common ones are table sugar or sucrose (composed of glucose and fructose) and lactose (the carbohydrate in milk containing glucose linked to galactose). There can be longer chains of these molecules, which we call polysaccharides. These chains are not only linked one to another in one line, but sometimes have other linkages that cause branching chains to be present. Starch is a family of such substances. Indigestible dietary fiber is also a type of polysaccharide; the human intestine does not contain the necessary enzymes to break down those specific branching points.

Whereas fat and carbohydrate are composed only of atoms of carbon, hydrogen, and oxygen, protein also contains another element, i.e., nitrogen. A protein is a chain of molecules called amino acids, and each protein differs in the sequence of the amino acids. There are about 20 amino acids; since any protein molecule can contain large numbers of them, the possible sequences are almost infinite. Some proteins function as building blocks for cells, whereas others are "enzymes," i.e., proteins that facilitate the occurrence of specific biochemical reactions.

In addition to these nutrients, the body also needs minerals and vitamins. Minerals are specific atoms or groupings of atoms, and they do not polymerize (form chains, as we have discussed for fats, carbohydrates, and proteins). Examples of minerals include sodium, potassium, chloride, phosphate, iron, calcium, magnesium, and zinc.

Vitamins are specific substances that the human body cannot manufacture but that are necessary cofactors for various biochemical processes. Because the human body does not manufacture vitamins, they must be obtained from other sources (usually plants).

We speak of vitamins as being water-soluble or insoluble. (The water-insoluble ones are described as being fat-soluble.) If you have ever mixed oil and vinegar in a salad dressing, this concept should be clear. If you simply pour oil (fat-based) and vinegar (water-based) together, one will layer out over the other; fat does not dissolve in water. Similarly, certain vitamins do not dissolve in water; these are vitamins A, D, E, and K. The other ones (all of the vitamin B's, folic acid, and vitamin C) will dissolve.

The final nutrient that we need, and one that we do not often think about, is water. At times the insufficient presence of water can become an important clinical problem.

Digestion and Absorption

As should be obvious from the above discussion, the nutrients (in particular, fat, carbohydrate, and protein) that we eat are large molecules in the form of chains of smaller molecules. These large molecules cannot be absorbed by the intestinal cells, and thus they have to be broken down ("digested") into their constituent pieces in the lumen of the intestine. Let us consider the role of each intestinal organ in this process.

Food is normally swallowed and passes through the esophagus into the stomach. The stomach is responsible for beginning the digestive process. Several actions occur at this location. First of all, the stomach begins to contract, and the food particles are broken up into smaller pieces by a grinding action. As part of this same activity, fat globules that are present are "emulsified" into solution (instead of one large globule, there are thousands of tiny ones) in much the same manner that tiny oil droplets form when the oil and vinegar mixture is vigorously shaken. The stomach will not discharge particles of solid food into the small intestine until they have reached a relatively small size.

The stomach also controls the rate of emptying of all nutrients. This emptying procedure is timed so that calories are introduced into the small intestine at a fixed rate, and the intestine is thus not overwhelmed by a sudden large load. (For example, dietary fat, which is calorie-rich on a gram-for-gram basis, slows gastric emptying.)

The stomach also secretes acid and an enzyme that facilitates protein digestion, called pepsin. However, it should be appreciated that pepsin and acid are not needed to accomplish normal food digestion. Actually, the primary role of acid in the stomach is to protect the host from microscopic organisms; the acid kills bacteria before they can gain access to the rest of the intestine and subsequently invade the body itself.

As the food particles enter the lumen of the small intestine, it is obvious that the long molecular chains are, by and large, still intact. (Remember that the food particles are macroscopic; molecules are orders of magnitude smaller and can only be seen with very sensitive electron microscopes.) The reduction of the size of the food particles, and the emulsification of the fat, simply provides more exposed surface area for the same volume. The biochemical digestion of the molecular chains is done with the assistance of specific enzymes that are secreted by the pancreas and enter the lumen of the small intestine at about the same time as the food arrives. One of the more important enzymes is pancreatic lipase, which separates two of the fatty acids from the triglyceride molecule.

Fat molecules, even as fatty acids, do not dissolve well in the intestinal fluid (which is water). To allow the fat to be packaged in microscopic particles that can then attach to the surface of the intestinal cells, the liver secretes bile salts. These bile salts spontaneously form "micelles," which are peculiar biochemical constructs with a fat interior (so the fatty acids and triglyceride molecules can be situated) and a water-soluble exterior (so that the entire particle can be "dissolved" in the aqueous intestinal fluid). Carbohydrates and proteins are water-soluble and do not need micelle formation for absorption.

It is only when the food chains are digested and in these smaller (microscopic) forms that the intestinal cell ("enterocyte") can absorb them. Assisting this process are enzymes on the luminal surface of the enterocyte, which further break down disaccharides (sucrose and lactose) and small chains of amino acids called peptides.

After the nutrients are absorbed, they are processed inside the enterocyte and then shipped out into the bloodstream (carbohydrates and amino acids) or lymph channels (fat). Since a number of potential toxins can also be eaten and potentially absorbed, the blood flow from the intestine is directed first to the liver (via the portal vein). The liver can then regulate what escapes into the systemic circulation.

Hence, the intestine is responsible for absorption. Amino acids and sugar molecules are usually taken up in the region of the small intestine which is nearer to the stomach ("proximal"). Fat, which has a more complicated digestive process (i.e., takes longer), is usually absorbed farther down ("distal") in the intestinal tract. Bile salts, which are needed for the fat absorption, are specifically absorbed after their work is done, at the end of the small intestine (called the terminal ileum) and transported back to the liver so they can be used again. This same region of the small intestine is the area where vitamin B_{12} is also specifically absorbed.

The primary role of the colon is to absorb water and salt (sodium chloride). The residue that reaches the colon is otherwise composed of cellular debris, indigestible fiber, and bacterial products. Some of the indigestible fiber can be metabolized by the bacteria in the colon; hydrogen and carbon dioxide can be produced, and this is the major reason why people who consume high-fiber diets often note increased flatulence.

Actually, any unabsorbed carbohydrates can be metabolized by the bacteria in the colon, producing, in addition to the above-noted gases, short chain fatty acids. This is of some importance in patients with gastrointestinal (GI) tracts that are incapable of absorbing nutrients normally, as these short chain fatty acids can also be absorbed by the colon and provide a source of energy for the body.

NUTRITIONAL PROBLEMS ASSOCIATED WITH INFLAMMATORY BOWEL DISEASE

Weight Loss

Loss of weight is a common problem in patients with a number of chronic diseases. Patients who are sick characteristically lose their appetite and reduce their intake of food. This is due largely to a normal physiologic response to illness, namely, the synthesis and release of a variety of chemicals ("cytokines") that have, as one effect, a suppression of appetite. (This is well recognized by anybody who has had a sick pet or child; when the pet or child feels better, his or her appetite returns.)

Perhaps with the exception of very severe weight losses, this loss of appetite and reduction of intake is simply a sign that something is wrong. Curiously, our society focuses on this aspect of illness, and well-meaning family members and friends are constantly urging patients to eat more.

I have often wondered why people stress this so strongly. The only answer I have been able to identify relates to my grandmother. She was always there when I got sick, chicken soup and hot tea in hand. I know she had long ago noted that when a person felt better he or she would then eat. I believe that she thought that if she saw me eat she could then be assured that I was feeling better, and this would be comforting to her.

In other words, my grandmother confused cause (the illness or its subsequent resolution) with effect (the suppressed appetite or its subsequent reappearance). As we will note later, a number of scientific studies have not been able to prove that increasing the nutrient intake to sick patients improves their outcome.

From our above discussion about normal physiology, it should be appreciated that most nutrient absorption occurs in the small intestine, so patients with only colonic disease should have all of those mechanisms still intact. In fact, patients with only colitis are far less likely to lose weight, and when the weight loss occurs it is usually in the setting of an acute flare of the disease (and the consequent cytokine release). Hence, the "nutritional problems" related to colonic disease are related to the loss of water and electrolytes (from the diarrhea) and, perhaps, loss of iron (from the blood loss).

Patients with Crohn's disease (CD) located in the small intestine can have specific problems that produce weight loss. The mucosal inflammation may be so severe that absorptive capacity is compromised; because of the large reserve, however, a great deal of intestine must be so involved. Occasionally, large segments of the intestine have been surgically removed, leaving inadequate absorptive surface to maintain normal weight.

Perhaps more often, the problem is due to the fact that eating stimulates gastrointestinal secretion and that these fluids cannot be adequately absorbed. The resultant diarrhea is unpleasant, and the patient avoids eating to avoid this symptom. The same food avoidance may occur in patients who have narrowing of the lumen of the intestine ("strictures"); eating may produce pain (if the intestinal flow is partially obstructed). Although many patients with CD can be shown to have malabsorption in challenge tests (in which a given amount of fat is taken in and the residual fat in the stool is measured), it is usually a reduced intake, rather the extra caloric loss, that accounts for most of the weight loss.

This is not to say that other specific malabsorption problems are never an issue. For example, a chronic bowel obstruction may predispose the intestine located just proximally to become dilated and overgrown with bacteria; these bacteria may interfere with some of the normal disgestive and absorptive functions. Another potential problem can arise in patients who have sclerosing cholangitis; in this condition, the bile ducts become narrower, and the amount of bile reaching the intestine is lessened, with a consequent decreased ability to form micelles. If the inflammatory process also involves the lymphatic system, there may be a problem conducting fat out of the enterocytes. Patients with IBD are not immune from developing lactase insufficiency. This is a normal condition in most non-Western populations; the small intestinal cells stop producing the enzyme that breaks down the milk sugar lactose (lactase). The unabsorbed lactose is carried to the colon, where the bacteria metabolize it (causing diarrhea and gas). Most such patients quickly recognize this condition and stop eating milk and milk products. It should be appreciated that such people are not "allergic" to milk; this is not an aberrant immune response, but rather a predictable consequence of an aging event. Furthermore, the calorie content of the dairy product is usually replaced by other foods, and weight loss is not usually an issue. Nonetheless, a flare of CD in the small intestine may also temporarily interfere with lactase generation, at least in those who are still producing it.

Other Nutrient Deficiencies

The best known nutritional complication of CD is vitamin B_{12} deficiency. As we have noted, that vitamin is specifically absorbed by receptors located in the terminal ileum (the last part of the small intestine). If that region is inflamed (or surgically removed), those receptors are lost. Again, there is an overabundance of receptors, so most patients with CD do not have this problem. It can be an issue when a large segment of that part of the intestine is lost.

Diarrhea can cause water and mineral deficiencies. This is certainly a problem with acute flares of the disease. It can also be an associated problem of various forms of malabsorption, as we have already seen. Some patients with disease of the terminal ileum lose their ability to absorb some of the bile salts. While the liver is able to increase the synthesis of those substances (so micelles can still form), the bile salts that escape into the colon can cause the colon to secrete water.

Oxalate is a substance found in a variety of foods (e.g., spinach, rhubarb, chocolate, cocoa, tea, beets, parsley, green beans). It is excreted in the urine. When too much of it is absorbed, crystals can deposit in the kidney and ultimately produce kidney stones or kidney failure. The amount of oxalate that is absorbed by the body is usually limited because free calcium in the intestinal tract binds to it and prevents its intestinal uptake. In the few patients who have true fat malabsorption (for our purposes, especially those who have had large amounts of their intestine removed but now have relatively inactive disease and good appetites), the free calcium can instead be complexed to fatty acids (because these fatty acids are not being absorbed). The oxalate can then be absorbed by the colon (if that organ is still present).

As might also be predicted, individuals with severe malabsorption will also not absorb all of the vitamins and minerals that they ingest. This is particularly problematic with the fat-soluble vitamins. If calcium is also restricted (e.g., patients with concomitant lactase deficiency and reduced milk product intake), the combination of vitamin D and calcium inadequacies can produce significant bone disease ("osteomalacia").

Anemia also occurs in patients with IBD. There are a number of reasons for this. Obviously, during the active phase of the disease, blood loss through the intestine is one factor. Furthermore, the same cytokines that suppress the appetite also act on the bone marrow to reduce the synthesis of new red blood cells. Over a longer period, iron deficiency can also develop, in particular in individuals who have restricted their food intake.

One of the classic manifestations of vitamin B_{12} deficiency is anemia. This is usually easily recognized because of the characteristic changes seen in the red and white blood cells.

Medications used to treat IBD can alter various metabolic processes. For example, Azulfidine can interfere with folic acid absorption. Osteoporosis, a disease of the bone in which the proteinaceous structural matrix (in which the calcium is embedded) is deficient, is a common long-term complication of corticosteroids. (This disease is different from osteomalacia, in which there is deficiency of calcium itself, although both diseases weaken the bone.) Cholestyramine, which is sometimes used to bind bile salts (and prevent the diarrhea described above), can also bind nutrients and make them unavailable for absorption.

NUTRITIONAL THERAPEUTIC CONSIDERATIONS

"The proof of the pudding is in the eating." —Miguel de Cervantes

Before beginning this section, we should develop some understanding about how physicians "know" things. Much of the traditional medical education process consists of learning what our mentors do and taking advantage of their experience and insights. This type of information can be classified as "expert opinion."

By incorporating expert opinion into our practice patterns without questioning how that opinion was developed, we essentially accept dogmatic rules. Not uncommonly, these rules turn out not to be true. (If you do not believe this, consider the medicinal practice of two centuries ago, when leeches and bloodletting were the answers to all diseases.)

A better way to know that a particular intervention is effective is to test it in a type of scientific study called a "prospective randomized controlled trial." In such a study, a population of patients is identified and, in a random fashion, each patient is assigned to a treatment group (in which the intervention is used) or a control group (in which it is not). At the conclusion of the trial, the outcomes of both groups are compared.

The principle of employing "randomized controls" is that only one variable is changed. This is certainly the intent of any controlled trial, but other types of controlled trials cannot change only one variable.

For instance, suppose we look at the charts of a group of patients and identify which ones did or did not have a particular intervention. While we could compare the ultimate outcomes in the two groups, our interpretation will be limited by the fact that more than one variable has been changed. Hence, we cannot definitively attribute any differences between the two groups to the variable of the receipt or nonreceipt of the intervention.

The second variable that has been changed is the reason why the intervention was or was not employed. For example, different doctors may have believed or not believed in it; in this case, the two groups of patients also had different physicians. Whatever the reason was for the intervention being used or not used, that reason constitutes a second variable.

For purposes of the following discussion, we will view the most powerful evidence for deciding whether a proposed therapy has efficacy as being data from prospective randomized controlled trials. On the other hand, from the perspective of evidence-based medicine (which is becoming the basis on which decision making is now occurring), expert opinion is considered to be the least reliable.

Does the Diet Cause Inflammatory Bowel Disease?

"Thy food shall be thy remedy." —Hippocrates

There is an old belief that patients with exacerbations of IBD should be treated by putting their intestinal tract at rest (i.e., not stimulating it), so that the intestine would not have to "work as hard." Of course, the intestine is not a muscle that fatigues, and thus the concept of hard work is probably inappropriate.

Nonetheless, a series of prospective randomized controlled trials has compared "bowel rest" (i.e., not feeding patients through their GI tracts, but giving nutrition intravenously instead) to feeding programs. In these studies (all in patients with CD), the outcomes were similar, suggesting that intestinal stimulation was not an important issue.

There is no good scientific evidence that has implicated any dietary factors in the etiology of ulcerative colitis (UC). We will, however, return in a moment to an interesting concept regarding the use of dietary fats in modifying the disease activity.

There has been some speculation that some component of the diet, in particular a dietary protein acting as an allergen or antigen (and producing an aberrant immune response in the intestine), is responsible for CD. The evidence for this is, however, indirect.

Perhaps the strongest argument for this hypothesis is an observation made a number of years ago by Virginia Alun Jones and her colleagues. They randomly assigned a group of patients who had CD in remission into one of two groups. One group received regular food; the other was placed on a challenge diet in which foods were introduced one at a time and any that led to symptoms were thereafter eliminated. Six months after starting the trial, none of the 10 given the regular diet were still in remission, but only 3 of the 10 randomized to the exclusion diet had had disease activation.

It should be noted that in the studies comparing feeding to bowel rest the feeding programs all employed commercially prepared, nutritionally complete (i.e., containing all of the necessary nutrients) formula diets, not simple food. Hence, even if there is some dietary antigen, the success of the feeding could have been due to the coincidental noninclusion of this (these) substance(s) in the manufactured diet. In fact, the formulas used in these trials were usually elemental diets, in which the nitrogen source was in the form of amino acids or small peptides. Any putative antigen is likely to be a larger molecule than those present in these feedings.

There have also been a number of randomized controlled trials in which patients with exacerbations of CD have been given either these formula diets or corticosteroids. Taken as a whole, the trials have shown that steroids are more efficacious (Griffiths et al., 1995).

On the other hand, the remission rates in the patients receiving the diets were somewhat higher than might be expected if the diets had no effect at all. Hence, these formulations may have some potential utility, at least as second line therapy. However, many of these diets have poor tastes and are not well tolerated by patients, especially if they are to serve as the only source of nutritional intake.

There is yet one more potential role of the diet in the pathophysiology of IBD. We have noted that triglycerides are the usual source of fat calories in the diet and that these substances are, in turn, composed of three fatty acids. Some of these fatty acids (called "omega-6 fatty acids") are precursors of the inflammatory mediators, or cytokines, that we discussed earlier. Hence, dietary fat may provide the substances that are converted by the body to molecules that produce the inflammatory response.

The fatty acids contained in fish oils are of a different biochemical structure in that they have different locations of the unsaturated bonds we discussed in the first section (the places where two wires held the atoms together). These are referred to as "omega-3 fatty acids" and they are precursors for other cytokines which, at least in laboratory models, produce a less severe inflammatory response. Hence, it is possible, at least in theory, that removing fat from the diet, or substituting omega-3 for omega-6 fatty acids, could be of benefit in reducing the amount of inflammation.

This is still a new concept and there is relatively little information available to support or refute it. One small randomized controlled trial by Middleton and co-workers (1995) suggested that the response of CD to elemental diets was poorer if the patients also received triglycerides containing long chain fatty acids. However, there were a number of confounding factors in this study that make reaching any conclusion difficult.

Several other small randomized controlled trials in patients with IBD have compared the use of fish oil supplements to standard fat supplements, with variable results. Although some of these investigators have concluded that there was benefit, if one carefully looks at the actual data, the differences are often limited to improvements in laboratory tests, not in symptoms. Furthermore, these studies did not include a true control group; based on our considerations above, the standard fat given the comparison groups may have caused harm. In summary, although the hypothesis is promising, there is inadequate proof for physicians to recommend low-fat and/or fish diets (or fish oil supplements) at this time.

There is no evidence at this time to suggest that fiber or its absence plays any role in IBD. By the time dietary fiber reaches the intestine it is in a liquid state. It is incorrect to view this substance as having "sharp points" that scratch the intestinal wall. In fact, many patients use exogenous fiber as symptom relief for (usually mild) diarrhea.

Nutritional Support as Therapy

"Health indeed is a precious thing, to recover and preserve which we undergo any misery, drink bitter potions, freely give our goods: restore a man to his health, his purse lies open to thee."—Robert Burton

Before discussing the specifics of nutritional support in patients with IBD, a point of clarification needs to be made. In the preceding section, we discussed specific nutrients that may potentially aggravate the inflammatory process (e.g., putative antigens or fats as precursors of cytokines). In this section, we will concern ourselves with a more generic issue, namely, the provision of nutrients to patients who are perceived to be, or are at risk of becoming, malnourished.

Among a group of patients with the same diagnosis, it is invariably true that those who lose more weight have poorer clinical outcomes. This observation has led many physicians to seek ways to increase the weight of their patients, believing that this would improve the outcome. (As we will see in a moment, this is actually a fallacious conclusion to draw from the observation, as it confuses cause and effect.)

One way to provide nutrition is by venous infusion; we are all familiar with the use of sugar solutions given intravenously. However, it should be remembered that a liter of the standard sugar solution (5% glucose) contains less than 200 calories of carbohydrate.

Hence, if one wants to give 2,000 calories, more than 10 L would have to be infused. For many patients this is too much volume to be easily tolerated. An obvious answer to this dilemma would be to increase the caloric concentration of the fluid; unfortunately, these "hyperosmotic" solutions, when infused into most veins, cause the veins to clot off.

In the 1960s it was found that a hyperosmotic solution could be infused into very large veins; the high blood flow diluted it before damage to the venous wall occurred. This technique became known as total parenteral nutrition (TPN). The ability to deliver large amounts of nutrients gave rise to a great deal of research and a medical industry. In fact, investigators went on to develop sophisticated techniques for using the intestinal tract to provide nutrients to patients who either could not (because of gastrointestinal problems) or would not (often related to the cytokine effect we discussed earlier) eat.

For our purposes, we will consider any artificial system of providing a liquid formulation containing the daily requirements of calories, a nitrogen source, vitamins, and minerals as "nutritional support." These liquids may be delivered into the veins ("parenteral nutritional support") or into the intestinal tract ("enteral nutritional support"). Enteral nutritional support can be provided through tubes (placed in the stomach or small intestine) or as special formulations to be swallowed. (We have already considered some of these formulations above.)

The popularity of nutritional support came from the belief that improving the weight loss (or other manifestations of malnutrition) would improve the outcome. The evidence for this came from the intuitive perspective that it was bad not to eat, from uncontrolled (or poorly controlled) reports of success (data equivalent to expert opinion), and from observations of the association between poor nutritional status and poor outcome.

We have already noted that the natural response to many illnesses is not to eat. This instinct has developed through the millennia and, like many other behaviors that are ingrained, it may have survival value. (For example, if fat makes things worse, it may be in the best interests of the injured organism to avoid taking any in.) We have also noted the dangers inherent in simply accepting expert opinion.

What about the third argument, the association between malnutrition and bad outcome?

It is known that association cannot prove causation. With regard to the example about weight loss, the fact that the outcome was poorer in those who lost weight does not mean that the weight loss caused the poorer outcome. An at least equally plausible explanation is that those who lost weight had more severe disease and that the poorer outcome was due to the presence of the more severe disease. (In this case, the presence of the malnutrition is simply a marker or messenger telling us that more severe disease is present; the ancients learned centuries ago that killing the messenger did not alter the message.)

Nutritional support has been evaluated in a number of prospective randomized controlled trials, and the data have been disappointing. In almost all of the studies, the investigators could not demonstrate that the clinical outcome was improved by providing parenteral or enteral nutritional support (Koretz, 1980, 1984) In fact, in some cases (cancer patients receiving chemotherapy or radiation therapy in particular), the parenteral nutrition may have even been responsible for an increase in infection rates (see statement by the American College of Physicians). These results are really not surprising. The therapy does not attack the disease per se, but only a symptom of it.

The randomized controlled trials of Dickinson et al. (1980) and McIntyre et al. (1986) compared the outcomes of patients hospitalized with acute colitis who were, or were not, given parenteral nutritional support. No differences were seen. One trial, in which patients with active CD were randomly given diet alone or diet with a formula supplement (Harries et al., 1983) found that the supplement did not improve the outcome; in fact, the patients had more diarrhea while taking it.

No one would argue against the proposal that patients with IBD should eat a nutritious diet. However, at this time, and based on the principles of evidence-based medicine, one cannot make an argument to advocate the further implementation of some program of nutritional support in most such patients, even if they have lost weight. (The real answer is to treat the underlying disease.)

On the other hand, there are two conditions when programs of nutritional support are probably of benefit. These are actually conditions in which the problem is directly related to a severe lack of nutrients, and hence the treatment is directed at the underlying "disease."

The first is the situation that is encountered when a growing child falls below the predicted height/weight curves. If left untreated, such children will usually become short adults. It has been demonstrated that normal growth can be achieved if enough nutrients are supplied. Although parenteral nutritional support can do this, it is an expensive undertaking. Studies have shown that the problem in such children is usually a reduction in food intake, as discussed above. Hence, if such children can be forced to eat, growth can be restored. At times this may require infusions of nutrients through tubes placed in the stomach. (This is often done at night, while the child sleeps.)

The second situation has been alluded to before and is usually the consequence of multiple surgeries, to the point where there is an inadequate amount of GI tract remaining to absorb the nutrients necessary to sustain life. (This is what is classically referred to as "short bowel syndrome." With regard to IBD, these patients universally have CD.) Such patients are threatened by starvation, and the supply of intravenous nutrients is the only option.

A variant of this scenario is the patient who has persisting severe disease (including complications such as fistulas) and who will not be able to eat for many weeks. It is likely that very few patients will survive many weeks of not eating; thus, parenteral nutritional support is appropriate.

These programs of parenteral nutritional support can be conducted in the home. The necessary techniques can be learned, and most patients do this for many years while pursuing otherwise normal lives. They usually infuse the nutrient solutions at night while sleeping, then disconnect during the day and go about their business. The only drawback is the expense, which is substantial. For a patient who needs complete parenteral nutrition (i.e., who absorbs virtually nothing), the cost of the program is on the order of $100,000 annually.

There are some patients with intermediate malabsorptive problems. Such individuals can survive with enteral feeding, but much of what they take in is not absorbed. We have considered this earlier, with regard to the creation and absorption of colonic short chain fatty acids (if that organ is in place) and the potential problem of oxalate. There are a few other issues that should be considered.

These patients often have severe diarrhea, and water and electrolyte deficiencies can occur. If the losses cannot be compensated for by drinking water, special rehydration formulas are available that facilitate sodium and water absorption.

When fatty acids are not absorbed by the small intestine, they are further metabolized by the colonic bacteria into substances that produce excess colonic water. The most famous of these substances is ricinoleic acid, a laxative otherwise known as castor oil. Hence, a low-fat diet may reduce the volume of diarrhea. In fact, the dietary long chain fatty acids can be partially replaced by medium chain ones. Medium chain triglycerides (which are triglycerides composed of medium chain fatty acids) are absorbed directly by the small intestine without the need for micelles and/or breakdown into fatty acids, and medium chain triglycerides are not precursors of these diarrheagenic substances.

Obviously, lactose may also be a problem, and this carbohydrate should, in general, be avoided. Vitamins and mineral supplements are often needed. Elemental diets, in which the various constituents have been broken down into smaller molecules, might have some theoretical benefit as well. However, in patients with severe intestinal disease, pancreatic secretion is still present, and the endogenous enzymes are thus still available to perform this function. Furthermore, these diets are difficult to consume orally, as the taste is unpleasant.

Obviously, patients whose main problem relates to strictures and subsequent symptoms of obstruction should avoid fiber. If the problem is severe, these individuals may even need to be placed on liquid diets.

SUMMARY

In this chapter, we have first looked at normal nutritional processes, namely, nutrients and their assimilation by the body. Energy comes in the form of carbohydrates and fat; dietary protein can also be used for this reason, but its constituent amino acids are more important when used to synthesize specific proteins for cellular structure and enzymes for cellular function. These substances are broken down into smaller molecules in the intestinal tract and are then absorbed by the intestinal cells. The other important components of the diet are water, minerals, and vitamins.

IBD presents the patient with a number of nutritional problems. Perhaps chief among these is weight loss, which is usually due to reductions in intake. This is, in turn, a consequence of either appetite loss (a cytokine effect) or the fact that the intake of food worsens other symptoms (in particular diarrhea and/or pain).

Other nutritional issues related to IBD are lactose intolerance and deficiencies, in particular vitamin and mineral deficiencies. The medications used to treat the disease can also have nutritional implications.

There is some soft and indirect evidence that particular dietary constituents may have pathophysiologic significance in the disease process, but these data are far from definitive. At this time, severe dietary changes (e.g., avoiding food with putative antigens or switching to a high-fish-oil diet) cannot be recommended.

Generally speaking, the generic use of nutritional support, with the intent of forcing patients to gain weight, also cannot be advocated at this time. However, such programs are appropriate for the few patients who are failing to grow or who have such severe malabsorption that normal feeding cannot sustain them.

SUGGESTED READINGS

Alun Jones V, Dickinson RJ, Workman E, Wilson AJ, Freeman AH, Hunter JO. Crohn's disease: maintenance of remission by diet. *Lancet* 1985;2:177–180.

American College of Physicians. Parenteral nutrition in patients receiving cancer chemotherapy (Position paper). *Ann Intern Med* 1989;110:734–736.

Dickinson RJ, Ashton MG, Axon ATR, Smith RC, Yeung CY, Hill GL. Controlled trial of intravenous hyperalimentation and total bowel rest as an adjunct to the routine therapy of acute colitis. *Gastroenterology* 1980;79:1199–1204.

Griffiths AM, Ohlsson A, Sherman PM, Sutherland LR. Meta-analysis of enteral nutrition as a primary treatment of active Crohn's disease. *Gastroenterology* 1995;108:1056–1067.

Harries AD, Jones LA, Danis V, Fifield R, Heatley RV, Newcombe RG, Rhodes J. Controlled trial of supplemented oral nutrition in Crohn's disease. *Lancet* 1983; 1:887–890.

Koretz RL. What supports nutritional support? *Dig Dis Sci* 1984;29:577–588.

Koretz RL, Meyer JH. Elemental diets—facts and fantasies. *Gastroenterology* 1980;78:393–410.

McIntyre PB, Powell-Tuck J, Wood SR, et al. Controlled trial of bowel rest in the treatment of severe acute colitis. *Gut* 1986;27:481–485.

Middleton SJ, Rucker JT, Kirby GA, Riordan AM, Hunter JO. Long-chain triglycerides reduce the efficacy of enteral feeds in patients with active Crohn's disease. *Clin Nutr* 1995;14:229–236.

CHAPTER 9

A GUIDE FOR PATIENTS AND THEIR FAMILIES TO MANAGE THE EMOTIONAL IMPACT OF INFLAMMATORY BOWEL DISEASE

Morton L. Katz

4544 Post Oak Place, #250, Houston, Texas 77027

How many people do you know who, on the eve of their marriage, would say to their spouse, "And most of all, I'm thankful that you have Crohn's disease?" Or, "I want to thank the Lord that your ulcerative colitis will bring experiences to our marriage and family life that few people will have the opportunity to partake of." The idea that any form of inflammatory bowel disease (IBD) would be hoped for, prayed for, counted on to strengthen family life is ludicrous.

The immediate emotional effect of learning that you have IBD is not a feeling of joy or of wanting to share the news with family and friends. Instead, you experience disbelief or maybe anger. You feel sorry for yourself, and you feel guilty for forgetting your blessings. You are afraid and perhaps confused. How normal! No sane person would be happy or relieved to hear that he or she will experience periods of time with cramps, diarrhea, and headaches for the duration. Thankfully, there is good news:

1. You can learn how to have a good life and adjust to the sporadic symptoms of IBD.
2. You are not alone; IBD does not affect only one person. Professional athletes, glamor queens, television stars, the son of a former president, Chris Gedney, Mary Ann Mobley, John York, Al Geiberger, and Marvin Bush all have led active and successful lives with IBD. There *are* ways to effectively manage IBD symtoms and their lack of predictability.
3. Without the certainty and security of knowing when the symptoms of IBD will appear, it is hard to make plans. How does one plan for what is not predictable? When you were a teen with a curfew, you knew what reaction to anticipate from your parents if you stayed out too late. You could decide whether it was worth the punishment to extend your good time. In college, you might occasionally drink and smoke too much, knowing exactly the price you would pay the next day. Now, the reality is that you cannot have security about how you will feel tomorrow or what you will be able to do next week. This chapter will teach you new self-management skills which address your decreased ability to anticipate the state of your health on a particular day.

4. What others can expect from you will be different. Of necessity you will be less dependable because you cannot foresee whether you will be able to participate in certain activities at a fixed future time. Your word about what you would do for or with others was your bond; as always, even though you are usually not this specific, the bond has always meant contingent upon.

5. What you need from others changes too. You must teach friends what you need from them, and your needs will include increased flexibility on their part. A component of your reality is that you are not going to feel really good or have complete freedom to go where you wish during periods of time of varying length. All of the activities you have participated in without a second thought will have to be considered carefully; you must change your expectations about your physical capabilities and accept that some physical limitations will exist for varying periods of time.

In this rush of feelings and thoughts, you may ask yourself: What did I do to cause this disease? Will I ever feel good again? Can I ever participate in activities I used to enjoy without worrying? Why is God mad at me? What am I going to do? The questions keep coming. It is necessary to make a major shift in the direction of thinking it through and away from focusing only on feelings when called on to make decisions regarding future activities.

1. The first thing you should do is obtain information about IBD. Consult the experts, books, people living with the disease. Although you need explanations and predictability, what you will get is "Sometimes," "Maybe," "It's hard to say," and "Well, sometimes it's this way and sometimes it's that way." It is hard to feel comfortable or informed with these types of responses. Nevertheless, your first goal should be to become better informed.

2. Your second goal is to get a clear sense of your options. Again, you are confronted with shades of gray. When you are worried, what you want is for someone to make the world more logical for you than it really is. Ask your doctor to make the information artificially black and white for the moment; later you will be able to tolerate the gray—the uncertainty—the reality.

In the long run there are three approaches to coping with IBD and how it impacts you:

1. You can try to change the disease. That is what the Crohn's and Colitis Foundation of America (CCFA) is all about: finding a cure for IBD. Your doctor can provide medications to moderate the symptoms and some forms of the disease are treatable with surgery. Please remember that you cannot change the effects of the disease with wishes or will power.

2. You can try to run away from the disease, to deny its existence. That approach is about as effective as trying to get away from a hurricane when you are in the middle of it.

3. You can ask yourself what you can change about yourself to manage living more realistically with IBD. You begin by changing what you can control: your expectations and your attitudes. Begin by clarifying your values, i.e., what really matters most to you in life. You are then in a position to analyze whether the lifestyle you have lived is the *only* way to live your values.

The troubling reality of IBD is that there is no way to escape from some forms of this disease, and the Foundation has yet to find a cure. The exciting reality is that there are ways to change your expectations and your attitudes, thus making life with IBD manageable and experientially enriched.

1. The first truth to remember is that any decision, situation, or consequence always has positive and negative aspects. You enjoy the entire late-night movie and the next day you are tired. You decide to buy a big-screen television or a new couch, so you have to put off buying something else you really want. You want a new computer with all of the latest upgrades, so you must postpone your vacation trip. Perhaps you can still take the trip on credit, but that means fewer dinners out, fewer movies or concerts for a long time. Most of us have never come to accept the reality that in life the grass really is, truthfully, greener in patches. We forget the "in patches" part. People tend to lose sight of the whole picture. Most of us look at part of the elephant and think we are describing the whole animal. Feelings that are not filtered through rational thinking direct us to look at life unrealistically. And the brain does not feel; it only uses logic. It is important to remember that there

is always a positive and a negative, and that appreciating the positive and negative aspects of anything is accomplished primarily by thinking, not by feeling.

2. Once you begin to use your head to deal with your disease, you will realize that no feeling lasts forever. It is indeed hard to remember that the immediate symptoms you are living with—the diarrhea, the fever, the cramping—will abate, as will the good feelings from that heavenly piece of pastry or from being completely relaxed after a great vacation. When you are in the throes of distress you can remind yourself (i.e., *think*) that these symptoms will pass, and that what you attend to, or focus on, really makes a difference. Ask yourself what role you want this time of distress, this pocket of discomfort, to play in your life. The reality is that, from the perspective of a 70-year-old person, the intensity of your distress which results from a canceled activity is significantly less.

3. What you feel is not the only important issue; it is what you do with your feelings that has an impact on you and those close to you. You will feel sick sometimes, and for those times you will need some books that you really want to read but rarely find time for; stationery for the letters you want to write but always put off; videos of movies that you'd like to see; you complete the list. Now is the time to treat yourself to interests you have never had the time to pursue: genealogy, gardening from seed and plant catalogs, becoming an expert in an area of interest. There is an interesting novel by Josephine Tey entitled *The Daughter of Time,* which chronicles the development of a passionate interest in the truth about King Richard III's place in history by a detective-inspector of Scotland Yard who is confined to a hospital bed. He is "climbing walls" until a clever friend ignites the inspector's curiosity to research and clarify the reality of Richard's role in history. You may not care about Richard III, but try to develop an interest that is compelling enough to occupy your mind during periods of enforced confinement. You can plan for the times you will have to hang around the house: Plan to make these times more interesting than they would be if you had nothing to do but dwell on your illness. (Hooray for the Internet!) If you do not plan, if you dig your head into the sand, then each time you

become ill you will have to reinvent the wheel. If you were making a long trip with small children, you would plan meticulously for diversions to keep them entertained while they were forced to be relatively immobile. You owe yourself the same degree of planning to make the time pass with the least possible feeling of enforced captivity. If you continue to behave in the ways you always have, without taking into account your new reality, you will be lucky if you don't end up feeling frustrated. If you plan purposefully, you will feel that you have some control over how your illness plays out. You will feel and have some control over how your time is occupied during flare-ups.

4. Although it is difficult, it is really important to separate your value as a person from what you do in your job, in your family life, in your social interactions, or in your physical activities. If these activities are restricted, you may feel *identityless*, and a realistic self-concept is vital to living successfully with IBD. I co-authored an executive coloring and activity book, in which there was a picture of a short, bald, rotund fellow wearing boxer shorts, looking in the mirror. In the mirror he has Speedo swimming trunks and an Olympic swimmer's physique. A realistic self-image, including what you do well and what you do not do well, will relieve a lot of immediate distress. You will relieve the distress that results from thinking of yourself as what you are not by thinking of yourself as what you are.

5. Be realistic and recognize that you do not like being included in the exclusive group of IBD sufferers. However, today it seems very difficult to feel sorry for yourself and to admit that you intensely dislike things in your life because you do have so much to be thankful for: decent clothes, food, a car, a home, and loved ones. We have all been taught from childhood to recognize how much better off than most other people in the world we are and to be ashamed of complaining or pitying ourselves. If you can just tolerate your normality, appropriately, it will not leave you feeling happy; however, allowing yourself some self-pity for a while will leave you calmer.

6. Another reality you can learn to deal with is that it takes time and many trials to learn how to live a complete life when IBD is a part of that life. However, in the present, you can make small

changes. You can learn what supplies go with you. You can learn to have systems in place for unexpected flare-ups at awkward times, such as when leaving for the airport or during a family vacation. As you experience the disease, you learn a little more each time about preparing for the subsequent flare-ups. It takes time to work out the systems that take care of you when you need a little more taking care of. No one writes in cursive beautifully the first time; no one gets on a bicycle or roller blades flawlessly without experience. If you take baby steps and measure these baby steps, you will not feel as if you are going nowhere. You will recognize that the steps become more secure with each experience.

Having suggested some initial adjustments in handling life with IBD, I would like to discuss some changes for the long run. I want to suggest certain steps that you can take that will substantially change how you structure and plan for yourself. Making adaptations in your lifestyle that allow for the stress, for the discomfort, for the lack of predictability that IBD poses is vital.

1. The first of these lifestyle changes is religion. It does not matter what form you subscribe to, but you might want to involve yourself in religion because religion helps put life's experiences, both enjoyable and unpleasant, in perspective. Religion gives you a context to healthfully understand that there can be new beginnings, that the past does not go away, and that you can live with what you wish had not occurred in your life. How you interpret what is happening around you is partially determined by how you view it. For example, a kid is playing baseball in her front yard and her mom and dad are watching her with the ball and bat. She takes the ball and throws it up, swings, and misses. The mother says to the father, "Honey, our 8-year-old can't even hit a baseball. I mean, can you imagine what her self-esteem is like to not even hit a baseball?" She throws it up a second time, swings, and misses. The father says to the mother, "I wonder if she contracted some of this learning disability stuff? You know it may even be in the water now." The girl throws up the ball the third time, swings, and misses. The parents rush up, and with a big smile on her face the girl says, "Great pitcher, eh?" The reality is that how you view

something greatly affects how you think and feel. Without faith it is very hard to have proper perspective on life.

2. You must not forget that it is crucial to feel sorry for yourself sometimes, in spite of the Judeo-Christian teachings that have taught us from childhood that self-pity is a sin. My reason for suggesting that self-pity can be healthy is that in balance it is normal not to like what one does not like. Most of us do not think about self-pity in that way, but it makes sense and provides clarity.

3. Adjusting to the reality that "life really is greener in patches" is a substantive part of the long-term changes that you need to make. Why? Because being realistic will help you appreciate what you have and what you do not have. Most of us are not very realistic in terms of our blemishes and beauty spots. A person bound to a wheelchair can either complain about not being able to run or can focus on being able to see the birds, smell the roses, and taste the strawberries. A blind person can focus either on not being able to see or on being able to hear conversation around him and to join in, to smell and taste a wonderful dinner, to walk, even if with some form of assistance. It is absolutely true that living with IBD is "icky." There is little that is positive about it. I do not believe that it "builds character." I doubt that it results in anything truly of value. However, what is true is that you can attend to what you cannot do, or you can attend to what you can do.

4. You can learn to sweat regularly. I would use the word "exercise" but I don't want to scare anybody. I do not mean running 5 miles at 3:30 a.m. every other day and pumping iron on the days in between. I am emphasizing the fact that if you exercise *a little* and relax *a little*, that is the way life is supposed to be. No system operates 24 hours a day without some down time. Planning exercise in a reasonable way with your physician and/or with someone who knows how to guide the exercising in a healthful way will make a huge difference in your sense of well-being and in your maintaining good physical health both for better emotional health and for your body's ability to cope better with IBD.

5. Next, it is important to begin in a purposeful and specific way to diversify how you are going to meet your needs. If you think about it, one person cannot realistically meet all your needs if

you have a flare-up that lasts for several weeks. It is vital to realize that your spouse cannot be your sole care giver. No matter how much a husband loves his wife, or a wife loves her husband, or a parent loves a child, no one person can continue cheerfully and efficiently to go through weeks with a loved one who feels terrible, smells terrible, and experiences discomfort most of the time, unless the care giver is able to get out and have some fun. What you need is to have other people involved in how you and your family live with the impact of IBD. It is like having an elderly family member whom you take turns helping. It is no different than parents' helping a young couple buy a new home. Society recognizes with "mother's day out" programs that even the most devoted mother benefits from a guilt-free day away from her small child or children. No one can give and give, and smile and be happy, and utilize prayerful forbearance constantly, while denying all personal needs and giving up all opportunities for relaxation and recreation. It is not realistic. With or without chronic illness, one person cannot meet all your needs in the long run. Some time ago I developed a program to teach children who learn more quickly than other children how to pick friends. Let's say you have a child of exceptional intelligence who is interested in astronomy or math or geology. He cannot pick a friend who likes baseball and expect that friend to spend hours studying the stars. You have to pick people in terms of considering realistically what you can ask of them, even if they are loved ones or friends.

What does it mean to build a good life and to account for the adjustments IBD symptoms require?

1. You need to learn to ask for what you want. You can learn to teach other people about your specific needs and how to fulfill them:
   a. "I want you to sit with me and do a crossword or jigsaw puzzle and not ask how I feel. I want you to focus on the puzzle and not on my facial grimaces. Please do not say that you hope I feel better. I may even complain about my day and all I want you to do is just go through the day and let me be grumpy and not feel good."

b. Do not assume that if you are feeling lousy the other person does not want to be around you. Making assumptions creates problems in marriages and friendships. Specific instructions take the pressure off a person who cares about you.

2. Make sensible comparisons to other people.

   a. As my wife and I walk out of a movie, she looks at a poster of Robert Redford with a longing glance and talks about his incredible acting. SHE IS NOT THINKING ABOUT HIS ACTING! I do not look like Robert Redford. Of course, he doesn't look like Robert Redford either except on the screen.

   b. My wife and I used to watch "Lifestyles of the Rich and Famous." It would be wonderful to have a 100-foot yacht anchored in the blue water in front of our 12,000 square foot third home. If I think I can have such a lifestyle on the salary of a psychologist, I will feel like I have the value of a penny waiting for change. Sensible comparisons help you live with IBD more reasonably.

3. You can learn to develop realistic expectations for yourself and others.

   a. Many people say to my wife, "You are so lucky to be married to Morton Katz. He is so sensitive, so caring, so interesting to talk with." After I am in the office for 12 hours, I don't want to talk to anyone. My empathy gauge is below empty. So, my wife and I have an understanding. One of us must indicate clearly when we really want to talk. The rest of the time I can be in the ozone.

   b. I teach a class at Methodist Hospital in Houston, Texas to help couples about to have their first child learn to change some of their short-term expectations of each other. These couples are not physically close in the ways they are at other times for several weeks prior to the birth of their child. Then they are not close in the usual ways for several weeks after the baby arrives. After many weeks of not being intimate, most men are not interested in reading poetry to their wives, and most wives are not in the mood for 3 to 7 hours of torrid love making. Having realistic expectations as concerns what will happen in the situation and how you might feel can help you plan for the future.

4. It is very important to have structure and predictability in the usual routines of your life because that will let you feel and indeed be in control. People feel in control when they can predict what will happen.
   a. If your husband clips his toenails and leaves them in the middle of the den next to his house slippers most of the time, but suddenly he picks up the toenails and the slippers, you will wonder what is up.
   b. If your husband or wife usually calls and says "Babe, I'm on the way home" and then arrives an hour and a half later, you are not concerned; but if one day the person came home at the exact time he or she promised, you would want to know what's up.
   c. Usually I take the garbage out after my wife has said something like, "Oh, honey did you remember the..." "Oh, yeah. I was just gonna do that." She and I both know I was not thinking about taking out the garbage. Three or four days ago I took it out without a prompt from her. And my wife saw me doing it and said, "What got into you?" I am not into garbage. The truth is that I was lucky enough to remember it that day, and the change in my behavior was startling to her, and disconcerting, even though it was positive.

It is very important that the routine of your lifestyle include plans for how to adjust when you have a flare-up. And I do not mean just toilet paper. I'm thinking about board games. I'm thinking about a plan B, i.e., that the kids know that at certain times they make their own lunches, they make their own beds, and they straighten their rooms. There is a plan in place that will allow life to continue in a reasonably normal way.

5. I think it is extremely helpful for a husband and wife to sometimes be a little stingy and self-centered in planning for IBD as part of their life. My wife and I work long hours. We share the responsibility associated with raising our daughter. When I need a break, I call my wife and tell her that I am going to the office supply store, turn off my beeper, and be there for about an hour. I love office supply stores. Why do I love them? Because you can get out of there with a sense that you can organize your

entire life: your money, your philosophy, your beliefs, your plans, your hopes. They have paper clips—big ones and little ones. And they are different colors. I mean, you can walk out of an office supply store completely calm. I do not spend enough time at home either with my wife, with my daughter, or with us as a family. We don't. It's impossible. But she supports me in this hedonistic behavior. Sometimes I even buy a fountain pen. The reality is that I do the same for her. You can live more realistically with your illness, whether there is a flare-up or not, if sometimes you are self-centered and hedonistic.

6. Sometimes you need to find somebody to listen to your woes who is not going to try to fix them. Where people who love you get stuck is that they want you to feel better and want you to be happier. If your husband or wife, mom or dad, brother or sister, or friend can't just listen, then call a friend and ask him or her to "just listen." "Woe is me" is the truth—sometimes.

The secrets to having a life that includes IBD and is rich in experiences are God and adjustability. If you think and act as you always have, then you can expect the results to be the same. If you learn to adjust, you can experience enhanced daily living. Please remember that we are talking about a process that you can only learn with the passage of time and the increased knowledge that comes from learning about yourself and your illness. You can effectively incorporate your IBD symptoms into how you plan and live your life.

CHAPTER 10

MEDICAL THERAPY

Mark A. Peppercorn

For many years, the drug therapy for inflammatory bowel disease (IBD) was limited to the use of sulfasalazine or one of several forms of corticosteroid. In recent years, the aminosalicylates based on sulfasalazine's structure have proved useful in both ulcerative colitis (UC) and Crohn's disease (CD). In addition, drugs that modulate the immune system such as 6-mercaptopurine (6-MP) and azathioprine have gained widespread acceptance in the therapy of IBD, and new immunomodulators such as cyclosporine and methotrexate promise to play a bigger therapeutic role in the future. Antibiotics, particularly metronidazole, are frequently administered to patients with CD. In addition to these agents, which have become the standard drug therapy of IBD, there are many additional drugs and therapeutic modalities under active investigation. Some of these have been studied in open trials in which both doctor and patient know that a single agent is being tested for its effectiveness. Others have been or are being investigated in controlled trials in which a potentially active agent is compared to an inert placebo in a study in which neither patient nor doctor knows which form of treatment the patient is receiving. This chapter reviews

Department of Medicine, Beth Israel Deaconess Medical Center, Boston, Massachusetts 02215; and Harvard Medical School, Boston, Massachusetts 02115

the current available information on both standard medical treatment and on those agents that show promise for the future.

THE 5-AMINOSALICYLIC ACID AGENTS

Sulfasalazine

Sulfasalazine (Azulfidine, Pharmacia and Upjohn, Kalamazoo, MI) was first introduced into clinical medicine in the late 1930s for the treatment of rheumatoid arthritis. The subsequent initial studies suggested the drug's efficacy in the treatment of UC, and eventually it became the most widely prescribed drug worldwide for the therapy of IBD. Controlled trials have established the effectiveness of sulfasalazine in active UC regardless of disease extent. The drug is particularly useful in maintaining remission in UC for indefinite periods of time. In addition, sulfasalazine will reverse flares of CD, especially when the colon is involved in the inflammatory process. Unlike the case with UC, sulfasalazine has not been shown to prevent relapses of CD in remission, nor does it prevent recurrence of the disease after operation.

For active UC and CD, the drug is usually begun at a low dose of 1,000 mg (one tablet 2 times per day), with a gradual increase in dosage over several days to 3 to 4 g per day. In rare instances, higher doses of 5 to 6 g per day may be prescribed. The drug often takes 3 to 4 weeks to achieve its full effectiveness, at which point the dose can be lowered. For patients with UC who achieve remission, a maintenance dose of 2 g per day usually is suggested. An extensive experience with sulfasalazine has determined that it is safe to begin or continue the drug during pregnancy, and it is not necessary to stop it when nursing begins.

Sulfasalazine consists of sulfapyridine (one of the first sulfa drugs) linked via an azo bond to (5-ASA), a compound related to aspirin. Sulfasalazine is partially absorbed in the upper intestine, and a portion is excreted in the urine, imparting a deep yellow color to the urine. The remainder of the drug traverses the intestine until it reaches the colon, where bacteria cleave the azo bond and divide the drug into its sulfa and 5-ASA components. The sulfa portion is largely absorbed and excreted in the urine, whereas the 5-ASA portion largely stays in contact with the colon and is excreted in the feces.

Side Effects

Although very effective in the treatment of IBD, the usefulness of the drug is limited by a high incidence of side effects. These include nausea, headache, and loss of appetite, which can usually be reversed by lowering the dose. Heartburn and indigestion are additional common side effects that may be avoided by the use of an enteric-coated form of sulfasalazine. Mild allergic reactions such as fever and rash can sometimes be overcome by a process of desensitization, in which very low-dose amounts of sulfasalazine are introduced, with a gradual increase in dose over several weeks. Mild degrees of lowered red and white blood cell counts may be reversed by lowering the dose, but severe forms require stoppage of the drug. Sulfasalazine interferes with folic acid absorption; however, this can be overcome with supplemental folic acid. Other more serious reactions that require stopping the drug include reversible infertility in males, exacerbation of colitis, hepatitis, pancreatitis, pneumonitis, and pericarditis. Most of the side effects can be attributed to the sulfa portion of sulfasalazine.

The observations on the breakdown and distribution of sulfasalazine suggested that the parent drug may be serving as a vehicle for delivery of an active component to disease sites. The 5-ASA portion seemed like the probable active agent because it alone remains in contact with the colon. This hypothesis, coupled with information on the side effects of the sulfa portion of the drug, led to the development of a new group of agents known as the aminosalicylates.

THE AMINOSALICYLATES

Topical Forms

In the initial study that confirmed the effectiveness of 5-ASA as a therapeutic agent, patients with UC involving the lower colon were given enemas containing either 5-ASA sulfapyridine or sulfasalazine. Both the 5-ASA and sulfasalazine agents, but not the sulfapyridine component, put the colitis into remission in over 70% of patients. Subsequent controlled trials have confirmed the efficacy of 5-ASA enemas in patients with active UC involving the rectum (proctitis) or both the rectum and the sigmoid colon (proctosigmoiditis). As with sulfasalazine, 5-ASA enemas also are useful at maintaining remission in such patients. A suppository form of 5-ASA effectively treats active ulcerative proctitis and will keep the proctitis in remission if used as maintenance therapy. Although these agents appear to be effective in patients with CD of the rectum and sigmoid colon, only limited studies have been done in such patients. 5-ASA in a foam form also has been tested and appears effective, but is not yet commercially available.

For patients with proctitis alone, 5-ASA suppositories, known generically as mesalamine (Rowasa, Solvay Pharmaceuticals, Inc., Marietta, GA) and containing 500 mg of the drug, are begun in the morning and at bedtime. Although effects may be seen within a few days with a decrease in bleeding, the full effect may take 4 to 6 weeks. At that point, the dosage can be reduced to nighttime only and then tapered to every other night or every third night as maintenance therapy. For patients with proctosigmoiditis, the 5-ASA or mesalamine (Rowasa) enemas are begun usually nightly, continued for 4 to 6 weeks and then tapered to a maintenance regimen of every other or every third night.

Oral Forms

Although the topical forms of 5-ASA are useful for patients with inflammation involving the lower colon, they are not effective alone for patients who have more extensive UC, or for the majority of patients with CD, which involves the small intestine and/or the colon above the rectum and sigmoid. In order to reach these areas, oral forms of 5-ASA had to be developed that would not be broken down by stomach acid or absorbed in the upper intestine before they would reach the lower bowel. Several forms of oral 5-ASA have been developed.

Slow Release Agents

One form of 5-ASA, or mesalamine (Asacol, Procter and Gamble, Cincinnati, OH), coats the drug with an acrylic resin, which dissolves as the pH of the intestinal fluid rises above 7. This allows delivery of the 5-ASA to the distal ileum and colon. Another form compresses the 5-ASA into microgranules that are coated with ethylcellulose (Pentasa, Hoechst Marion Roussel, Kansas City, MO). The 5-ASA is released throughout the small intestine and colon.

Azo-Linked Agents

Olsalazine (Dipentum, Pharmacia and Upjohn, Kalamazoo, MI) joins the 5-ASA to itself via an azo bond and, like sulfasalazine, requires bacterial cleavage in the colon for release of the active free 5-ASA moiety. Balsalazide (Colazide), which is still under study and not commercially available, links 5-ASA to an inert polymer, also through an azo bond, requiring bacterial release to free the 5-ASA. Both of these agents target 5-ASA release to the colon.

Controlled trials have shown the efficacy of oral forms of mesalamine, olsalazine, and balsalazide in active UC regardless of disease extent and in maintaining remission in UC. It is not clear as to whether any of these agents is any more effective for these conditions than sulfasalazine itself. The oral mesalamine agents appear to be effective in active CD even when the small intestine is involved and show promise in maintaining remission in CD, especially for patients with ileitis. Some exciting early studies suggest that the oral mesalamine agents may help prevent or delay recurrences of CD following resection and anastomosis.

For active UC and active CD, these drugs often have to be used in high doses to achieve maximal effect. The dose ranges include 2.4 to 4.8 g for Asacol (400 mg per tablet), 2 to 4 g for Pentasa (250 mg per tablet), and 1.5 to 3 g for Dipentum (250 mg per tablet). Once the therapeutic effect is achieved, usually in 3 to 4 weeks, the dose can be lowered and drug continued in a maintenance fashion (Table 1).

Side Effects

As was anticipated, eliminating the sulfa portion from sulfasalazine has enabled over 80% of patients intolerant or allergic to sulfasalazine to take either topical or oral aminosalicylates without ill effects. As with sulfasalazine, these agents appear to be safe in pregnancy and nursing, although there is only limited experience with the drugs under these circumstances. However, side effects have been reported with the aminosalicylates, and at times the same reaction seen with sulfasalazine has been noted with the aminosalicylates, thus implicating the 5-ASA as the offending agent. Adverse reactions include anal irritation with the 5-ASA enemas (perhaps related to the sulfite carrier), rash and fever, exacerbation of colitis,

TABLE 1. *5-Aminosalicylic Agents*

Drug	Dosage	Indication(s)
Topical		
Mesalamine enema (Rowasa)	4 g	Active proctosigmoiditis [a]Remitted proctosigmoiditis
Mesalamine suppository (Rowasa)	500 mg	Active proctitis [a]Remitted proctitis
Oral		
Sulfasalazine (Azulfidine) (enteric-coated and plain)	500 mg	Active ulcerative colitis Remitted ulcerative colitis [a]Active Crohn's disease
Mesalamine (Asacol)	400 mg	Active ulcerative colitis Remitted ulcerative colitis [a]Active Crohn's disease [a]Remitted Crohn's disease
Mesalamine (Pentasa)	250 mg	Active ulcerative colitis [a]Remitted ulcerative colitis [a]Active Crohn's disease [a]Remitted Crohn's disease
Olsalazine (Dipentum)	250 mg	[a]Active ulcerative colitis Remitted ulcerative colitis
Balsalazide (Colazide)	500 mg	[a]Active ulcerative colitis [a]Remitted ulcerative colitis

[a]Not an FDA-approved usage.

diarrhea (especially with olsalazine), pancreatitis, pneumonitis, and pericarditis. Unlike sulfasalazine, the 5-ASA agents do not cause male infertility, and anemia and leukopenia are rarely seen. However, a very small number of cases of kidney damage associated with the use of mesalamine have been reported.

CORTICOSTEROIDS

Corticosteroids were first used for patients with UC in the 1940s and have become a mainstay of therapy for IBD patients since that time. Depending on the extent and severity of the inflammatory process, patients are treated with either topical forms or oral forms, or are given the steroid by injection or intravenously (parenterally).

Topical Forms

Steroid suppositories, foams, and enemas are effective in treating active ulcerative proctitis and ulcerative proctosigmoiditis. Although less well studied in CD, they can be effective as well when the CD involves the lower colon. Once the process goes into remission, however, topical steroids, unlike the 5-ASA products, are not effective at maintaining the proctitis or colitis in remission.

For patients with proctitis, hydrocortisone suppository or foam (Cortifoam, Schwarz, Wilwaukee, WI) is administered nightly or twice daily, with a response usually noted within 2 to 3 weeks. Similarly, for proctitis or proctosigmoiditis, the hydrocortisone enema (Cortenema, Solvay, Marietta, GA) will be prescribed on a nightly or, occasionally, twice-daily basis and continued until a therapeutic response is noted. The topical steroid can then be tapered to an every-other-day regimen for an additional week or two and then stopped, since there is no benefit in long-term therapy once a remission is achieved. Moreover, with prolonged administration of topical steroids, the side effects so common with oral and parenteral steroids can be expected.

Oral Forms

Prednisone, methylprednisolone, and prednisolone are the usual oral forms of corticosteroid given to patients with disease that extends beyond the reach of topical agents or with a clinical picture serious enough to warrant therapy with these potent drugs. Most patients who are given oral steroids will have already received some form of a 5-ASA agent and either not have done well with it or have been intolerant to it. Oral forms of steroids have been shown to be effective in active UC and in active CD involving either the small bowel or colon. As with topical steroids, there is no benefit of oral steroids in maintaining remission in either UC or CD. Therefore every attempt to taper and stop the drug is made once the desired therapeutic benefit is achieved.

Prednisone (Deltasone), the most commonly used oral steroid, is usually begun at a dose of 40 to 60 mg/day, depending on the severity of the inflammation and the weight of the patient. This dose is usually maintained for 10 days to 2 weeks, at which time a response can be expected. The drug will then be tapered by 5 to 10 mg/week, with the goal of complete withdrawal of the steroid. Prednisone as well as topical steroids can be used safely in pregnancy and nursing. Unfortunately, a sizable proportion of patients who achieve benefit from the prednisone at higher doses begin to have a flare of their UC or CD as lower doses are reached. Such steroid-dependent patients are the ones most at risk for the long-term steroid side effects.

Parenteral Forms

Patients with severe and at times fulminant UC or CD will almost always require hospitalization. In addition to receiving intravenous fluids and electrolytes and, often, intravenous nutrition, such patients usually are treated with high doses of steroid delivered intravenously or occasionally intramuscularly. Such therapy can reverse and calm the disease process in 50% to 70% of patients, thus avoiding the need for surgery.

For patients entering the hospital already on an oral steroid, either hydrocortisone (SoluCortef) at a dose of 300 mg/day, methylprednisolone (SoluMedrol) at a dose of 48 to 60 mg/day, or prednisolone at a dose of 60 to 80 mg/day will be administered. If significant improvement is not seen within 10 days to 2 weeks, then in most instances surgery becomes an important consideration. Once improvement is achieved, patients can be switched to an oral form of steroid, which is then gradually tapered and hopefully stopped, as in the less severely ill patients. Patients who enter the hospital but have not been recently on oral steroids may receive corticotropin, or adrenocorticotropic hormone (ACTH), a hormone that stimulates the patient's own adrenal glands to produce and release cortisol, a form of steroid related to hydrocortisone. There is some evidence that for such patients with severe UC, ACTH may be more effective than standard steroid preparations.

Rapidly Metabolized Steroids

For many years, patients with asthma and allergic rhinitis have been treated with topical forms of steroids that have potent anti-inflammatory actions, but that are rapidly cleared from the bloodstream by passage through the liver. This rapid metabolism prevents the buildup of the drug, thus eliminating most of its side effects. These agents are now being studied in patients with IBD, and the early results of such studies are very promising. Budesonide is the agent under the most intense investigation. Budesonide enemas appear to be as effective as 5-ASA and hydrocortisone enemas for patients with ulcerative proctosigmoiditis. Moreover, a delayed release oral form of budesonide appears to be of benefit in patients with active Crohn's ileitis and ileocolitis when the cecum and ascending colon are involved. Patients with CD who achieved remission from symptoms on budesonide had a delay in the relapse of their symptoms if continued on the drug. Currently, these agents are not commercially available in the United States.

Side Effects

Although very effective at treating active UC and CD, adverse reactions to steroids are common. Insomnia, alterations of mood, and a voracious appetite as well as night sweats and altered glucose metabolism are side effects that may occur early, especially at high doses of drug. With more prolonged usage, even at lower doses, moon facies, acne, the development of a fatty hump at the base of the neck, and excessive hair growth are often noted. Cataracts, muscle weakness, osteoporosis, and hypertension are usually sequelae of long-term steroid usage. Osteonecrosis of certain joints, especially the hip, is rare and usually seen in patients who receive very high doses of drug for a prolonged period.

IMMUNOMODULATORS

6-Mercaptopurine and Azathioprine

6-MP (Purinethol, Glaxo Wellcome, Inc., Research Triangle Park, NC) and azathioprine (Imuran, Glaxo Wellcome, Inc., Research Triangle Park, NC) alter the immune system by inhibiting the effects of T-helper lymphocytes (CD4 cells), thought to play a prominent role in the inflammatory process in IBD. Azathioprine is metabolized by the liver to 6-MP, and the drugs can be used interchangeably. Both have been shown to be useful in active CD with regard to improvement in overall symptoms, healing of fistula, and allowing the dose of steroids to be lowered. They also are effective in maintaining remission in CD. Recently, these agents have been shown in controlled trials to be efficacious in active UC, regardless of disease extent, and in preventing relapses of UC in remission.

Both 6-MP and azathioprine are usually reserved for patients who have failed to respond to treatment with 5-ASA drugs and steroids, are intolerant to these agents, or are dependent on steroids to maintain a reasonable state of function often at the price of steroid side effects. Most patients can begin on an initial dose of 50 mg/day, which can be increased to a maximum 1.5 mg/kg/day for 6-MP and 2.5 mg/kg/day for azathioprine, depending on the response. These drugs, unlike 5-ASA agents and steroids, often take 3 months to have their full effect, although there are some patients who respond more quickly and some individuals may take 6 to 9 months to show an effect. Once a desired therapeutic effect is achieved, these agents are usually continued for a minimum of 1 to 2 years. A recent study suggested that continuing these drugs for 4 years was the optimum time to decrease the incidence of relapse after withdrawal of the drug. Although it is advisable to stop these agents during pregnancy, there is increasing evidence that 6-MP and azathioprine can be safely used during pregnancy without fear of adverse effects on the fetus. Since there is no information available with regard to nursing, it is best to stop these drugs during the periods of nursing.

Side effects

Although the concept of altering the immune system seems frightening to patients, 6-MP and azathioprine have proven to be remarkably safe agents. Reversible short-term side effects have been noted in less than 10% of patients and include allergic reactions such as fever and rash, nausea and headache, pancreatitis, and bone marrow depression with lowering of the white blood cell count in particular, as well as hepatitis. Long-term side effects occur in less than 2% of patients and primarily are severe infections and lowering of the white blood count. Rarely, lymphoma has been reported in IBD patients on these agents.

Cyclosporine

Cyclosporine suppresses the immune system by interfering with the effects of CD4 cells on inflammation. It has proven an invaluable agent in preventing rejection in organ transplantation. The administration of cyclosporine has been effective in inducing remission in patients with CD refractory to other agents. However, the relapse rate on withdrawal of cyclosporine often is rapid, and low doses of the drug are not useful in maintaining remission. Similarly, persistent Crohn's fistulas may heal after a short course of intravenous cyclosporine but frequently recur as the drug is withdrawn. Cyclosporine enemas have been tried in ulcerative proctosigmoiditis with variable success, although a controlled trial did not demonstrate efficacy. An important role for cyclosporine appears to be emerging in patients with severe UC unresponsive to high-dose intravenous steroids. In a controlled trial, over 80% of such patients responded within 1 week to treatment with intravenous cyclosporine compared with no response to placebo therapy. The long-term impact of cyclosporine on the eventual course of these patients is still being studied. Cyclosporine should be avoided during pregnancy although successful pregnancies in women on the drug have been reported.

Side Effects

A variety of short- and long-term adverse effects have been reported with cyclosporine. These include excessive hair growth, numbness of the hands and feet, seizures, opportunistic infections, hypertension, and kidney dysfunction. Blood levels of the drug must be monitored carefully during its administration.

Methotrexate

Long used in the treatment of psoriasis and rheumatoid arthritis, methotrexate has more recently been studied in patients with IBD. Open trials suggest efficacy for the drug in both active and remitted CD and UC, although the benefits of long-term use in both disorders were somewhat limited. In a recent placebo-controlled trial, methotrexate was effective in inducing remission in patients with active CD who had been on a dose of prednisone greater than 20 mg/day prior to the trial. In those patients who had been on a dose of prednisone less than 20 mg/day, the drug was no more effective than placebo. In a recent placebo-controlled trial, methotrexate was not of benefit in a group of patients with active UC. There are no controlled trials yet reported on the use of this drug for IBD patients in remission.

Side Effects

Adverse effects in these trials to date have been limited but include nausea, abnormalities of liver enzymes, lowered white blood cell count, and a potentially serious form of pneumonitis. This agent should not be used in pregnancy or nursing.

Potential Other Agents

There are early promising open trials and small controlled trials using innovative therapies which modulate the immune system. These include the administration of monoclonal antibodies to CD4 cells to patients with UC and CD, intravenous immunoglobulins to UC and Crohn's patients, a monoclonal antibody to tumor necrosis factor to Crohn's patients, and interferon to a group of Crohn's patients. For several years, there has been advocacy for a process called T-cell apheresis, during which numerous T cells are removed from the circulation. Open trials of this technique suggest that it may be of use in inducing remission in active CD. A recent controlled trial showed no benefit of T-cell apheresis in preventing relapses of CD, although patients on therapy were able to have their steroid dose lowered. The future utility of this expensive procedure is not clear. Finally, hydroxychloroquine (Plaquenil, Sanofi Pharmaceuticals, New York, NY), used to treat malaria and thought to affect the way intestinal cells process foreign substances, showed promise in open trials in UC but did not appear to be any more useful than a placebo in a controlled trial. Further studies with this drug may be forthcoming.

ANTIBIOTICS

Metronidazole

Metronidazole (Flagyl, Searle and Co., Chicago, IL) is effective in inducing remission in active Crohn's colitis and in treating the fistulas, sinus tracts, and abscesses that occur in CD involving the perineum. There are no studies as to its role in maintaining remission in CD, but one study suggests that it could delay recurrences of disease up to 1 year if given as a course of therapy immediately after surgical resection. It has not appeared to be useful in active UC although it should be considered in unresponsive relapses of UC, since undetected *Clostridium difficile* infection responsive to metronidazole may be associated with such relapses. One study did suggest that metronidazole may be as effective as sulfasalazine in maintaining remission in UC. In addition, metronidazole is useful in treating pouchitis after the ileoanal anastomosis and pouch procedure for UC.

For patients with Crohn's colitis and pouchitis, the drug is usually begun at a dose of 10 mg/kg/day and may be increased to 20 mg/kg/day for nonresponders. An effect is usually seen within 1 month, and after 6 to 8 weeks of treatment the drug is stopped. For pouchitis, a 10-day course of treatment using similar doses is usually beneficial. For patients with perineal CD, higher doses for longer periods often are required to achieve a positive result, and the relapse rate on withdrawal of therapy is high.

Side Effects

Adverse reactions to metronidazole often limit its usefulness. These include nausea, headaches, loss of appetite, a metallic taste, "furry" tongue, and the development of yeast infections. These are reversible upon withdrawal of the drug. Numbness of the hands and feet is usually seen only at higher doses of the drug, but the discomfort may linger long after the drug is stopped.

Ciprofloxacin and Other Broad-Spectrum Antibiotics

Ciprofloxacin (Bayer Corporation, West Haven, CT), one of the new quinolone antibiotics, has been effective in open trials of active

Crohn's ileitis, ileocolitis, and perineal disease. It has also been used effectively in conjunction with metronidazole in CD. In a recent controlled trial, the drug was more effective than placebo in a group of patients with refractory active UC. Its use follows a long history of anecdotal reports of the utility of other antibiotics in CD. These include ampicillin, tetracycline, and cefalexin. Whether these antibiotics affect undetected bacterial pathogens or, more likely, block the effects of the standard bacterial flora on the inflammatory reaction is not clear. Hopefully, in the near future, controlled trials of antibiotics in CD will establish more firmly a role for these agents.

Antituberculous Agents

The isolation of a tuberculosis-like organism from the tissues of several patients with CD has led to trials of therapy utilizing drugs directed against tuberculosis. Although the data are somewhat conflicting, a controlled trial in active CD showed no efficacy for a combination of such agents. In contrast, a controlled trial of several antituberculous drugs in CD in remission showed the drugs to be more effective at maintaining remission than placebo. Finally, clarithromycin, a new agent that is effective against both tuberculosis-like organisms and standard bacteria, induced prolonged remissions in a small group of patients with active CD. Antituberculous therapy with multiple drugs in CD is currently not commonly used, and more studies will be needed before there is widespread acceptance of such therapy.

LIPOXYGENASE INHIBITORS

The breakdown of a fatty component of cell membranes (arachidonic acid) by an enzyme called lipoxygenase leads to the production of certain chemicals that promote intestinal inflammation. It is thought that sulfasalazine and other 5-ASA agents may work in part by inhibiting the effects of lipoxygenase. Fish oil, another inhibitor of this enzyme, has been shown to have limited effectiveness in active, but not remitted, UC. However, it may take up to 18 fish oil capsules per day to achieve an effect. Although this agent is very safe, it can impart a fishy odor to the breath. A new enteric-coated slow release form of fish oil was better than placebo in prolonging remissions for patients with CD. These agents can be considered as safe alternatives to more conventional therapies.

NICOTINE

Smoking appears to protect patients from developing UC and may improve symptoms. In contrast, smoking seems to worsen the course of CD. In follow-up of these observations, transdermal nicotine patch (Nicoderm) has been studied in two controlled trials in active UC and improved symptoms significantly more than placebo. The agent was not useful, however, in prolonging remissions in UC. Side effects were common, especially in nonsmokers, and included lightheadedness, nausea, and sleep disturbances. Nicotine patch may be a useful addition to the therapy of active UC in patients not responsive to standard agents. However, the safety of its long-term use has to be questioned given the addictive potential and possible adverse effects that are clearly associated with smoking.

ANTIDIARRHEAL AGENTS

Antidiarrheal agents such as loperamide (Imodium), diphenoxylate with atropine (Lomotil, Searle and Co., Chicago, IL), codeine, and deodorized tincture of opium can be invaluable adjuncts to other therapy in patients with chronic stable diarrhea. Their use at bedtime can be particularly helpful in allowing a good night's sleep. Such agents need to be avoided in severely ill patients because their use may precipitate toxic dilatation of the colon in both UC and CD. Bulk agents such as psyllium (Metamucil, Konsyl) and methylcellulose may be helpful in thickening up watery stools. They also can be of use in patients who have associated irritable bowel–like symptoms with a sense of incomplete evacuation.

Cholestyramine (Questran, Bristol-Myers Squibb, Princeton, NJ) is especially effective in controlling diarrhea in patients with CD who have had an ileal resection. In such patients, bile acids, which are poorly absorbed because of the loss of part of the ileum, cause the colon to produce increased amounts of fluid, causing a watery diarrhea. By binding the bile acids before reaching the colon, cholestyramine can decrease the frequency and looseness of the stools. It is usually administered as a powder by mixing one scoop or one packet in juice taken 1 to 3 times per day.

ANTICHOLINERGIC AGENTS

Painful spasms of the intestine in patients with IBD may be relieved by anticholinergic medications, which temporarily block the transmission of nerve impulses in the bowel. There are a variety of such drugs, including propantheline (Pro-Banthine, Roberts Pharmaceutical Corp., Eatontown, NJ), dicyclomine (Bentyl, Hoechst Marion Roussel, Kansas City, MO), and hyoscyamine sulfate (Levsin, Schwarz Pharmaceuticals, Inc., Milwaukee, WI). Since these agents do not selectively work on the intestine, side effects are common and include dry mouth, visual disturbances, and urinary hesitancy and retention. As with antimotility agents, their use should be avoided in seriously ill patients because of the risk of toxic dilatation.

PSYCHOTROPIC AGENTS

The emotional stress that frequently accompanies IBD can be helped by the judicious use of antianxiety agents such as diazepam (Valium, Roche Pharmaceuticals, Manati, Puerto Rico) and oxazepam (Serax, Wyeth-Ayerst, Philadelphia, PA). For patients with more serious emotional disturbances, antidepressants such as amitriptyline (Elavil, Zeneca Pharmaceuticals, Wilmington, DE) and doxepin (Sinequan, Pfizer Inc., New York, NY) often are indicated. These agents also have anticholinergic properties that may affect bowel function. In addition to or in place of such agents, behavior modification techniques have been increasingly utilized. Similarly, support groups and educational material as provided by the Crohn's and Colitis Foundation of America can be invaluable in allaying patient concerns and providing emotional support (see Chapters 9 and 14).

MISCELLANEOUS AGENTS THAT SHOW POTENTIAL BENEFIT

A variety of therapies in addition to those described previously have given promising results for IBD patients either in small controlled trials or open studies. These include cromolyn sodium, lidocaine gel, bismuth, and short chain fatty acids given as enemas to patients with proctitis and proctosigmoiditis. Allopurinol, dimethylsulfoxide, penicillamine, and vitamin E all inhibit the production of forms of oxygen derived from white blood cells involved in the inflammatory reaction and believed to be injurious to intestinal cells. Limited studies of these agents in UC and CD have shown benefit. Similarly, subcutaneous heparin and factor XIII, substances important in blood clotting, have appeared promising in a few patients with UC. Finally, hyperbaric oxygen has been reported to be effective in several patients with very severe refractory perineal disease. More investigations of these agents will be necessary before their routine use in IBD patients can be advised.

DRUGS THAT MAY EXACERBATE COLITIS

Nonsteroidal antiinflammatory drugs (NSAIDs) can be of great benefit in treating the arthritis associated with IBD. Unfortunately, these agents may at times cause flares of colitis and in themselves can cause a colitis that is hard to distinguish from IBD. Therefore, the potential benefit of these drugs has to be weighed against this possible risk. Other drugs that can cause colitis include gold, used to treat rheumatoid arthritis, and retinoic acid, an acne treatment. Oral contraceptives have been associated with the development of both CD and UC, but the literature has given conflicting results as to whether the association of birth control pills and IBD is real. It is reasonable to consider stopping the birth control pill if the IBD began shortly after its institution and is not responding as expected to standard therapy. A wide variety of antibiotics including penicillins, cephalosporins, and clindamycin can cause a colitis that can be confused with flares of IBD (*Clostridium difficile* colitis). In addition, a number of drugs can cause diarrhea without exacerbating the IBD itself. These include magnesium-containing antacids, quinidine, and antibiotics.

APPENDIX 1. *Management of active ulcerative colitis*

Symptom	Medication	Dose
Mild to moderate		
disease	5-ASA suppository	bid or tid
Proctitis	Cortisone foam	hs or bid
Distal colitis	4-g 5-ASA enema	qhs
	Hydrocortisone enema	qhs
	Sulfasalazine	2.0–4.0 g po/day
	Mesalamine	2.0–4.8 g po/day
	Olsalazine	2.0–3.0 g po/day
Left-sided colitis and	Sulfasalazine	2.0–4.0 g po/day
pancolitis	Mesalamine	2.0–4.8 g po/day
	Olsalazine	2.0–3.0 g po/day
	Sulfasalazine/oral	
	5-ASA plus	
	5-ASA enemas/steroid	
	enema	
	Prednisone	40–60 mg po/day
Severe active disease		
On steroids recently		
	Prednisolone	60–80 mg IV/day
	Methylprednisolone	48–60 mg IV/day
	Hydrocortisone	300 mg IV/day
	Cyclosporine (in steroid	2–4 mg/kg IV/day
	failures)	
No steroids recently	ACTH	120 U IV/day
Toxic megacolon	Intravenous	
	corticosteroids	
	Broad-spectrum	
	antibiotics	
Chronic active disease		
(steroid refractory)	6-Mercaptopurine	50 mg po/day up to 1.5
	Azathioprine	50 mg po/day up to
		2.5 mg/kg po/day
	Methotrexate	10–15 mg po/week 25
		mg IM/week

bid, twice a day; tid, three times a day; hs, at bedtime; qhs, every hour of sleep; po, orally; IV, intravenously; IM, intramuscularly.

APPENDIX 2. *Maintenance of remission in ulcerative colitis*

Symptom	Medication	Dose
Proctitis	5-ASA suppository	500 mg every night to every 3rd night
Distal colitis	5-ASA enemas	4 g every night to every 3rd night
Left-sided colitis and pancolitis	Sulfasalazine	1–2 po/day
	Mesalamine	1.2–2.4 g po/day
	Olsalazine	1 g po/day
	Sulfasalazine/oral 5-ASA	1–2.4 g/d
	plus 5-ASA enema	4 g every night to every 3rd night
Steroid-dependent colitis	6-Mercaptopurine	50 mg po/day up to 1.5 mg/kg po/day
	Azathioprine	50 mg po/day up to 2.5 mg/kg po/day
	Methotrexate	10–15 mg po/week

APPENDIX 3. *Medical management of active Crohn's disease*

Symptom	Medication	Dose
Mild-to-moderate active disease	Topical hydrocortisone	
Oral lesions	Sucralfate	
Gastroduodenal disease	H_2 blocker, omeprazole	
	Sucralfate	
	Prednisone	40–60 mg po/day
Ileitis	Mesalamine	2–4.8 g po/day
	Ciprofloxacin	500 mg po bid
	Prednisone	40–60 mg po/day
Ileocolitis and colitis	Sulfasalazine	3–4 g po/day
	Mesalamine	2–4.8 g po/day
	Metronidazole	10–20 mg/kg/day
	Prednisone	40–60 mg po/day
Perineal disease	Metronidazole	10–20 mg/kg/day
	Ciprofloxacin	500 mg po/bid
	6-Mercaptopurine	50 mg/day up to 1.5 mg/kg day
Fistula	Metronidazole	10–20 mg/kg po/day
	6-Mercaptopurine	50 mg/day up to 1.5 mg/kg/day
Severe active disease		
Ileitis/ileocolitis/colitis Focal peritonitis	Broad-spectrum antibiotics	
No peritonitis	Prednisolone	60 mg IV/day
	Methylprednisolone	48–60 mg IV/day
	Hydrocortisone	300 mg IV/day
Chronic active disease (steroid refractory)	6-Mercaptopurine	50 mg/day up to 1.5 mg/kg po/day
	Azathioprine	50 mg/day up to 2.5 mg/kg po/day
	Methotrexate	10–15 mg po/week 25 mg IM/week

APPENDIX 4. *Maintenance of remission in Crohn's disease*

Symptom	Medication	Dose
Ileitis	Mesalamine	1.2–2.4 g po/day
Ileocolitis and colitis	Sulfasalazine	2–3 g po/day
	Mesalamine	1.2–2.4 g po/day
Perineal disease	6-Mercaptopurine	50 mg/day up to 1.5 mg/kg po/day
Postoperative recurrence	Mesalamine	2–3 g po/day
	Metronidazole	10–20 mg/kg/day
Steroid-dependent	6-Mercaptopurine	50 mg po/day up to 1.5 mg/kg po/day
Crohn's disease	Azathioprine	50 mg po/day up to 2.5 mg/kg po/day

SUGGESTED READINGS

Bitton A, Peppercorn MA. Medical management of specific clinical presentations. *Gastroenterol Clin North Am* 1995;24:541–558.

Feagan BG, Rochon J, Fedorak FN, et al. Methotrexate for the treatment of Crohn's disease. The North American Crohn's Study Group. *N Engl J Med* 1995; 332: 292-7.

Greenberg GR, Feagan BG, Martin F, et al. Oral budesonide as maintenance treatment for Crohn's disease: a placebo-controlled, dose-ranging study. *Gastroenterology* 1996;110:45–51.

Hanauer SB. Inflammatory bowel disease. *N Engl J Med* 1996;334: 841–848.

Lichtiger S, Present DH, Kornbluth A, et al. Cyclosporine in severe ulcerative colitis refractory to steroid therapy. *N Engl J Med* 1994;330:1841–1845.

Peppercorn MA. Antiinflammatory agents. In: Targan SR, Shonahan F, eds. *Inflammatory bowel disease: from bench to bedside.* Baltimore: Williams & Wilkins, 1994;478–486.

Prantera C, Zannoni F, Scribano MB, et al. An antibiotic regimen for the treatment of active Crohn's disease. A randomized controlled clinical trial of metronidazole plus ciprofloxine. *Am J Gastroenterol* 1996;91:328–332.

Present DH, Korelitz BI, Wisch N, et al. Treatment of Crohn's disease with 6-mercaptopurine. A long-term, randomized, double-blind study. *N Engl J Med* 1980; 302:981–987.

CHAPTER 11

SURGICAL THERAPY FOR INFLAMMATORY BOWEL DISEASE

Guy R. Orangio

GENERAL OVERVIEW

People with inflammatory bowel disease (IBD) can develop complications that will require surgical therapy. Surgery is classified as elective, urgent, or emergency. The preoperative and postoperative management of people with IBD is the same for Crohn's disease (CD) or ulcerative colitis (UC). The preoperative concerns are nutritional status, current medications, operative plan, psychological preparedness, risks and benefits of the intended procedure.

The preoperative nutritional status of people with IBD has been affected by chronic diarrhea, loss of appetite, pain, nausea, vomiting, and malabsorption. This leads to weight loss and malnutrition, which affects the immune system and the normal healing process. In ideal

Department of Medicine, Saint Joseph's Hospital of Atlanta, and Medical College of Georgia, Atlanta, Georgia 30342

situations, preoperative enhancement of nutritional status with either oral elemental diets or central hyperalimentation may lessen postoperative infection and time to recovery. However, when complications of IBD are severe, then urgent or emergency surgery is necessary.

Current medications utilized for the treatment of IBD suppress the natural immune system and thereby decrease the inflammatory response of the disease. Corticosteroids and immune modulators (6-mercaptopurine, azathioprine, cyclosporine) are the mainstay of medical therapy today. The surgeon must have a thorough understanding of the systemic affects of these medications, and an absolutely meticulous surgical technique must be utilized to diminish the possibility of postoperative complications. Corticosteroids should not be decreased during the immediate preoperative or postoperative period. A gradual tapering dose should be utilized postoperatively with careful physician monitoring during that time.

Many people with IBD are highly motivated and well educated about their disease and want to participate in the decision making process for their intended surgery. The risks and benefits of the intended operation must be explained openly and clearly. The overall benefits of the operation must be discussed so that a thorough understanding of the expected outcome is not greater than the reality of the true outcome. One of the greatest preoperative fears people have is that of being left with an ostomy after surgery. If an ostomy is required, then preoperative consultation with an enterostomal therapist is essential for marking and thorough explanation of its management. In addition, a preoperative visit from a United Ostomy Association trained visitor can be helpful. These visitors are generally matched by type of ostomy, reason for ostomy, age, and sex, and can answer personal questions regarding life with an ostomy. The surgeon could also offer to the patient a list of previously operated individuals with whom to speak about their surgical experience and current lifestyle. The person should be directed to the local chapter of the Crohn's and Colitis Foundation, as well as the United Ostomy Association of America, for information on support groups. People to people communication is essential to a better understanding of the surgical experience. I believe that much of the preoperative anxiety can be alleviated by an open, honest discussion of the intended procedure, possible complications, and realistic outcome.

The immediate preoperative preparation for people undergoing bowel surgery is a mechanical cleaning of the gastrointestinal tract with laxatives (Colite; Nippin Chemiphar) and enemas. This will decrease the amount of feces in the bowel, thereby decreasing the possibility of postoperative infection. Oral and intravenous antibiotics are utilized in combination with the mechanical bowel prep to decrease the chance of wound infection. Sometimes people with IBD are very anemic and may require a blood transfusion preoperatively. Intravenous fluids are started in the hospital prior to the operation. If an ostomy is required, then the enterostomal therapist or the surgeon can mark the abdomen for the optimal location for the intended ostomy. It is difficult enough for a person to have an ostomy, but one that is improperly located is absolute misery.

Even when all preoperative measures have been taken and the surgical procedure performed carefully, postoperative complications can occur. The possibility of hemorrhage, infection (abdominal or wound), or anastomotic leak (site of reattachment of the bowel) can occur and must be treated rapidly and effectively. The team approach to management of people with IBD is exemplified by surgical therapy.

SURGICAL THERAPY IN CROHN'S DISEASE

Two thirds to three quarters of patients with CD will need surgery at some time during their lives, and it is important to understand why an operation might be indicated. People who do require surgery should realize that it is not for cure of their disease but for a better quality of life. Some operations are required for serious complications, others performed for elective indications. CD affects the entire gastrointestinal tract from the mouth to the anus (Fig. 1).

Complications requiring urgent or emergent procedures are hemorrhage, perforation of the bowel, intestinal obstruction, abscess or fistula formation, cancer of the colon or small bowel, or toxic megacolon (dilatation and loss of muscle tone in the colon) (Fig. 2). Elective surgery may be indicated because medical treatments have failed to control symptoms such as pain, weight loss, fever, extreme fatigue, growth failure, or the side effects of these medications may be intolerable.

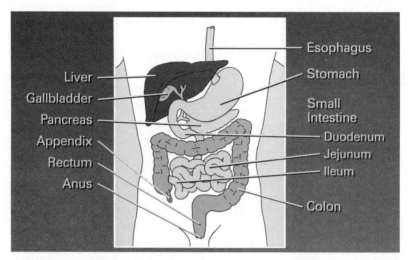

FIG. 1. Normal gastrointestinal anatomy.

The surgical therapy of anorectal disease in people with CD is very specialized. Abscess, fistula, and fissure formation of the rectum and anal canal are very painful and debilitating conditions. Treatment should be directed at maximum relief and minimal damage to the anal sphincter muscles (the muscles of fecal control) (Fig. 3).

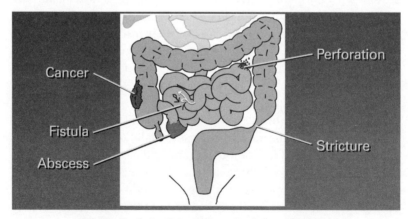

FIG. 2. Crohn's disease. Intestinal complications.

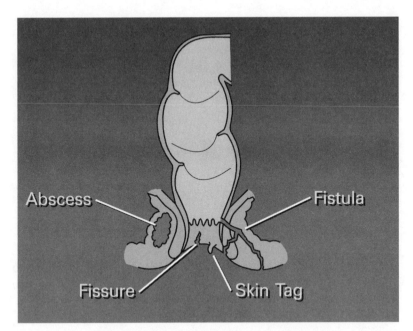

FIG. 3. Crohn's disease. Perianal problems.

The most common indications for emergency surgery are perforation of the bowel, massive hemorrhage, cancer of the bowel, or toxic megacolon (very unusual today). A bowel perforation can occur suddenly with severe abdominal pain, tenderness, fever, chills, vomiting, and even shock. The most common site of perforation is the distal ileum (small bowel). Massive gastrointestinal hemorrhage can occur from Crohn's colitis or an ulceration of the ileum. The symptoms of large amounts of black and foul-smelling stool (melena), gross rectal bleeding, dizziness, weakness, and shock are classic for gastrointestinal hemorrhage. Toxic megacolon is not very common today because of better medications and a team approach to management. The symptoms of toxic megacolon are tender distended abdomen, fever, chills, and tachycardia (high heart rate). Medical management is utilized for at least 48 hours, and if the patient is unchanged, then surgery is performed. The finding at surgery is usually a perforation of the colon with an associated abscess.

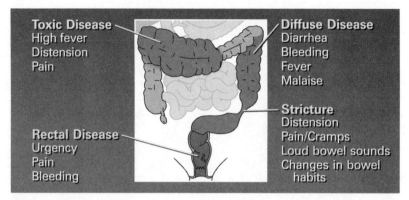

FIG. 4. Features of inflammatory bowel disease of the colon. Crohn's colitis.

The most common complication of CD is bowel obstruction and this can be either complete or partial. The symptoms are crampy abdominal pain, nausea, vomiting, intolerance to food, weight loss, and inanition. A classic finding of CD is "skip areas" in the bowel, i.e., areas of normal bowel interposed with areas of disease. This can occur in either the small or large intestine (Figs. 4 and 5). The cause of obstruction is chronic inflammation and scarring of the diseased

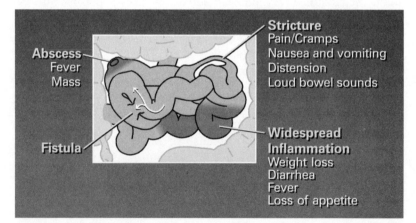

FIG. 5. Features of inflammatory bowel disease of the small bowel. Crohn's colitis.

bowel; an area of narrowing forms causing minimal passage of intestinal contents leading to crampy abdominal pain, nausea, and vomiting. The crampy abdominal pain is a reaction of the normal bowel in its attempt to force the intestinal contents through the narrowed segment. This increased activity causes dilatation and pain. This vicious cycle can lead to perforation of the bowel.

The type of surgical procedures in people with CD depends on the location of the diseased segment of bowel. The most important aspect is surgical conservation of bowel. A portion or a segment of diseased intestine that is causing symptoms can be removed. If it is a smaller segment with a stricture, a strictureplasty can be performed. This technique of widening the strictured area without removing that segment of bowel thereby allows passage of the intestinal contents (Fig. 6). This procedure is not recommended for colonic disease with associated obstruction. However, the use of conservative surgery in colonic disease is an alternative approach. This is for highly selected people with symptomatic disease limited to one section of the colon. A partial intestinal resection with anastomosis is when a diseased portion of intestine is removed and the remaining ends of the bowel are rejoined

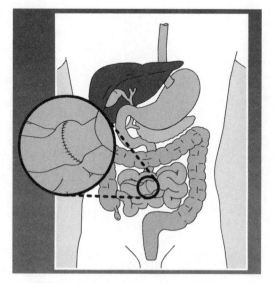

FIG. 6. Crohn's disease. Strictureplasty.

together to restore intestinal continuity (Fig. 7). This type of surgery does not result in construction of an ostomy. There are various names for surgical resections and this depends on which part of the intestine is removed and anastomosed (connected) together. For example, when a portion of the ileum (small intestine) is removed along with the cecum (a portion of the large intestine), the procedure is called an ileocolic resection with ileoascending colon anastomosis (the parts of the small and large intestine that are joined together). When a portion of the colon is removed, then a colon-to-colon or colon-to- rectum anastomosis is formed. When the entire colon is removed and the ileum is attached to the rectum it is called a total abdominal colectomy with an ileal rectal anastomosis. When the entire colon and rectum are removed and a permanent ileostomy is constructed, the operation is called proctocolectomy with end ileostomy (Fig. 8).

When the small intestine is involved with multiple small areas of stricture formation causing partial or complete obstruction, these skip areas can be managed with strictureplasty.

The surgical approach to anorectal fistulas, abscesses, and fissures is complex and should be combined with medical therapy for

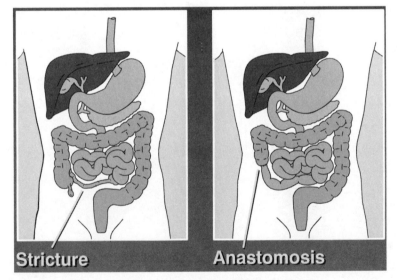

FIG. 7. Crohn's disease. Partial intestinal resection.

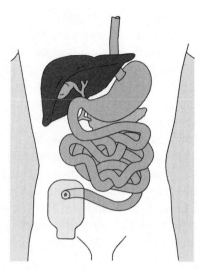

FIG. 8. Crohn's disease. Proctocolectomy and permanent ileostomy.

optimal results. The surgeon must have a thorough understanding of anorectal anatomy and physiology. The signs and symptoms of perianal disease are pain, bleeding, redness (erythema), hardness (induration), and drainage of foul-smelling thick pus. Controlled surgical drainage is favored over spontaneous drainage because this may allow for treatment of the associated fistula or fissure. This also allows for less damage to the anal sphincters.

Complex intestinal fistulas are common in people with CD. These fistulas or connections from the intestine to another intestine or organ can be very debilitating and socially stressful. Women can develop small bowel or rectal connections to the vagina, causing fecal drainage through the vagina. When there is an ileal vaginal fistula, the operative approach is resection of the involved small bowel with anastomosis of the small bowel. If there is a rectovaginal fistula, then a transanal (through the anus) repair is most effective. This is called an endoanal advancement flap, using a flap of the rectum as a patch to cover the fistula tract.

Sometimes a temporary ostomy is necessary to allow for adequate healing of the site. There are many reported cases of small bowel fistula to the urinary bladder, kidney, stomach, duodenum, colon, or the abdominal wall. A combination of medical and surgical therapy gives the most permanent results to the patient.

CD can affect the stomach causing ulceration and obstruction that may require specialized surgery of the stomach or duodenum. Surgical therapy of people with CD is highly technical and considerable experience is essential to allow for conservation of bowel and an improved quality of life.

The recurrence of symptomatic CD at the line of surgical resection is 20% at 2 years, 30% at 3 years, and approximately 50% at 5 years. After proctocolectomy and ileostomy, the recurrence rate is less than 20% at 5 years. Most people with recurrent CD after surgical resection respond well to medical therapy. In fact, only 40% to 50% of them require a second surgical resection. Approximately 10% to 30% require a third procedure for recurrent symptomatic CD.

SURGICAL THERAPY IN ULCERATIVE COLITIS

UC is limited only to the colon and rectum. This limits the types of surgical procedures that can be performed on people who require surgical therapy (Fig. 9). UC involves the rectum (proctitis), or the

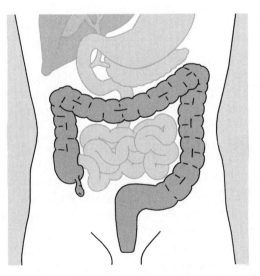

FIG. 9. Normal gastrointestinal anatomy of the colon and rectum.

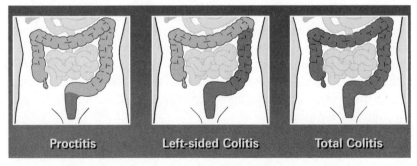

FIG. 10. Ulcerative colitis. Small intestine not involved.

left side of the colon (proctosigmoiditis), or the entire colon and rectum (pan or universal colitis) (Fig. 10). The most important finding is that the rectum is always involved with UC. If there is rectal-sparing disease then CD must be strongly considered. Colonic complications of UC that require surgical intervention for cure of the disease is present in 25% to 40% of patients. The indications are hemorrhage, toxic megacolon, perforation, mild stricture, severe dysplasia (premalignant), and cancer of the colon or rectum (Fig. 11). Some patients do not respond to medical therapy and cannot be tapered from the medications without developing a flare-up of their colitis. The type of surgical procedure indicated will vary with the

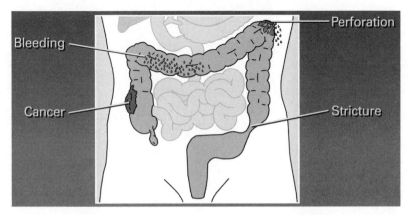

FIG. 11. Ulcerative colitis. Colonic complications.

condition of the patient and the experience of the surgeon. When a person has massive hemorrhage, perforation, fulminant colitis, or toxic megacolon, then surgery must be performed quickly. Usually, the procedure of choice is removal of the colon with an end ileostomy, leaving the rectum in place. Then, several months later, the patient may have a definitive operation to address the residual rectum and ileostomy.

There are three recommended surgical procedures for UC. The first procedure is proctocolectomy (removal of the colon and rectum), with salvage of the anal muscles (sphincters) by construction of a new rectum (neorectum) from the distal small bowel (reservoir or pouch) and a temporary ileostomy (Fig. 12). The loop ileostomy is closed after 6 weeks. The more common name for this procedure is the ileal pouch–anal anastomosis (J-pouch). This procedure usually requires two stages (two operations); however, recently in selected people, a one-stage procedure was safely performed. This is a procedure that can be performed in all age groups. After the operation, people average six to eight bowel movements per day. The consistency of the stool varies, but is mostly soft, almost putty-like.

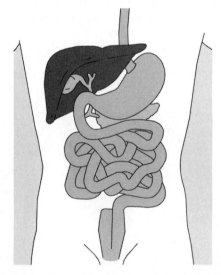

FIG. 12. Ulcerative colitis. Ileal pouch anal anastomosis.

As with any operation, there are short- and long-term complications. Approximately 7% to 10% of people with J-pouches will require conversion to a permanent ileostomy. The reasons for this are CD of the pouch, chronic pelvic infection, and overall poor tolerance of the pouch. The most common long-term complications are small bowel obstruction and pouchitis (a nonspecific inflammation of the pouch). Almost 20% of patients develop small bowel obstruction secondary to adhesions. Most respond to medical therapy, intravenous fluids, and bowel rest. However, some require reoperation to release the bowel from the scar tissue. This does not mean an ostomy or removal of the J-pouch. Pouchitis is a nonspecific inflammation of the pouch that occurs in 30% to 40% of individuals with J-pouches. It can be acute or chronic with associated systemic affects of malaise, fever, diarrhea, anemia, weight loss, loss of appetite, and even arthralgias (joint pain). It can usually be managed with oral antibiotics (metronidazole or ciprofloxin). The therapy usually is for 3 to 6 weeks. Some people may require topical medications applied in suppository or enema suspensions (Rowasa, Cort enemas).

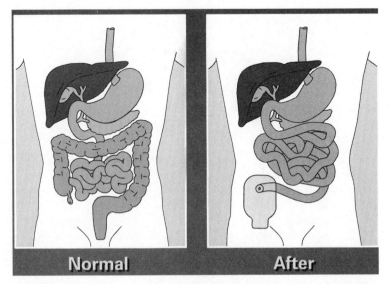

FIG. 13. Ulcerative colitis. Proctocolectomy and permanent ileostomy.

The operation that was the gold standard for the surgical treatment and cure of UC until the advent of the J-pouch is proctocolectomy and ileostomy (Fig. 13). This is still an excellent operation and is widely recommended to some patients who want only one operation and are emotionally ready to live with a permanent ileostomy. The operative technique is removal of the entire colon and rectum including the anal muscles with construction of an end ileostomy.

The third procedure is really for selected patients with "indeterminant colitis" involving only the colon and not the rectum. This type of colitis is so named because the pathology and the clinical findings are not specific for either Crohn's colitis or UC and the most important feature is sparing of the rectum. This is a very safe operation that involves removal of the colon and attaching the small bowel to the rectum (total abdominal colectomy with ileorectal anastomosis) (Fig. 14). This is a good choice for patients with this type of disease pattern because it does not leave them with a permanent ileostomy or possible failed J-pouch. Over the next 5 years, the "true disease" process will manifest, so that the definitive operation can be

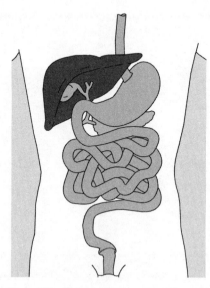

FIG. 14. Ulcerative colitis. Total colectomy and ileorectal anastomosis.

performed. The real disadvantage of this operation is that some type of medical therapy will be required for maintenance of the rectum.

The use of a continent ileostomy in people with Crohn's colitis is absolutely contraindicated. It is a highly technical operation that has a high reoperation and failure rate. It can be recommended to people who have a permanent ileostomy and want to attempt a new lifestyle or people with ostomy appliance problems. Any person who wants to convert to a continent ostomy should seek the opinion of several experts before going ahead with this procedure.

The surgical therapy of people with UC is very positive and is a means for cure of the disease. Although no procedure is perfect, a better quality of life is achieved and maintained.

MINIMALLY INVASIVE SURGERY FOR IBD

Since 1991, laparoscopic surgical techniques have been applied to bowel surgery. Selected people with CD or UC who are candidates for urgent or elective procedures may be candidates for laparoscopic surgical procedures. For example, people with ileal colic CD without infection can have an ileocolic resection with anastomosis utilizing laparoscopic techniques. More experienced laparoscopic surgeons can perform more complex procedures for ileal vaginal or urinary bladder fistulas. For people with UC who require proctocolectomy, an ileostomy and construction of a J-pouch are also candidates for this approach. The major advantages of laparoscopic or minimally invasive surgical techniques is less postoperative pain, less time in the hospital, and a quicker return to normal lifestyle. The complication rate should be the same as that for the standard open procedure.

Surgical therapy for people with IBD is part of the continuum of care. It should not be considered the last resort but part of the management of a very complex chronic disease.

CHAPTER 12

LIFE AFTER SURGERY

Tracy L. Hull

Surgery for any problem puts the patient in an uncomfortable situation. First, there is a fear of the unknown and of trying to determine exactly what procedure is needed. Second, there is the question of how the outcome will permanently affect one's life. Usually, when dealing with inflammatory bowel disease (IBD), patients feel like their back is against the wall and they have no choice but to go ahead with the surgery. In an effort to control their anxiety, most learn as much as possible about the operation and what to expect. This chapter is designed to go one step further and discuss things to expect after the surgical recovery. Since IBD is a diverse condition, postoperative highlights of the more common procedures will be discussed. I will focus on questions I am frequently asked, and some of my comments may reflect biases that stem from my education and experience at the Cleveland Clinic.

Department of Colorectal Surgery, The Cleveland Clinic Foundation, Cleveland, Ohio 44195

ULCERATIVE COLITIS

The continent ileostomy

Initially all patients with colonic IBD underwent a total procto-colectomy (removal of colon and rectum) and permanent ileostomy when surgery was necessary. With the knowledge that ulcerative colitis (UC) only affected the colon and did not recur after resection in the small bowel, efforts were made to eliminate the traditional ileostomy, which required an external collection bag for stool. One of the first pioneers was Dr. Nils Kock who in 1969 reported on the continent ileostomy. With this procedure the colon and rectum are removed and a pouch is constructed from the small bowel. The outflow of stool from this pouch is controlled by a "nipple valve" that is made by infolding a segment of the small bowel. This nipple valve prevents stool from escaping until a tube is inserted into the pouch to drain it. The internal pouch is connected to the abdominal wall via a flat stoma, and a small dressing may be worn over the stoma. When the pouch is full a catheter is passed through the stoma (intubation) into the pouch and the stool is drained (Fig. 1).

This procedure is currently not the operation of choice for patients needing surgery with UC. However, it remains an excellent option for patients who have previously had their sphincters (the muscles that control having a bowel movement) removed, have sphincter damage, or have a failed pelvic pouch. Patients frequently inquire as to how they will know to drain their pouch (i.e., with the tube) because postoperatively the tube is left in place continually while the surgical area heals. Then the tube is removed and a scheduled time of intubation is started. This means that on a strict time schedule the pouch is intubated and emptied, and gradually the time between intubations is increased. Eventually most patients learn to sense when their pouch is full by a pressure sensation over the pouch. Some describe it as "rectal pressure" on the abdomen. After a steady state is achieved most patients intubate their pouch 2 to 8 times daily.

This is a very complicated surgery and one of the reasons it is not popular is the potential long-term problems that may occur with the nipple valve. Slippage or prolapse of the nipple valve may occur in up to one third of patients with the need for revisional surgery. Additionally, patients are encouraged to have some dietary limitations.

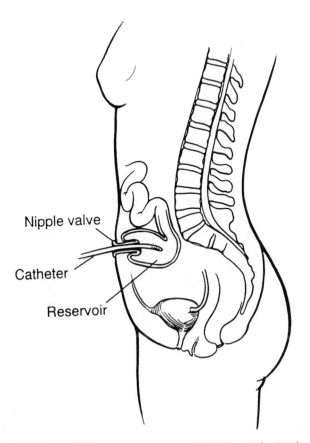

Nipple valve

Catheter

Reservoir

FIG. 1. The continent ileostomy involves an internal pouch attached to the abdominal wall with a flush stoma. The nipple valve allows this pouch to be continent. Stool is evacuated when a tube is passed through the stoma into the internal pouch. (Reprinted with permission from Hull TL, Erwin-Toth P. The pelvic pouch procedure and continent ostomies: overview and controversies. *J Wound Ostomy Continence Nurs* 1996;23:163.)

Essentially anything that will not evacuate through a tube (roughly the size of an adult's index finger) is avoided. This includes many raw vegetables and fruits that do not fully digest or that come to the pouch in their firm, nondigested consistency. Thinner stool aids in evacuation of the pouch.

Pouchitis (inflammation of the pouch) is another entity that can affect patients with any type of internal pouch for their entire life with the pouch. This condition usually is manifested as excessive pressure, pain, and cramping over the pouch. It may be accompanied by fever, malaise, or arthralgia. The cause of this condition is not known. It is usually treated by a short course of medication, with metronidazole being the most popular. This condition can recur after treatment.

The Pelvic Pouch

In the 1950s surgeons experimented with operations to eliminate a permanent stoma in patients with UC. There were many setbacks along the way and it was not until 1978 that Parks and Nicholls paved the way for the modern ileoanal pelvic pouch procedure. Today this is the preferred operation for patients with UC.

In a review of our patients who have undergone a pelvic pouch procedure (Fazio et al., 1995) 93% felt their functional results and quality of life were good to excellent. The average number of bowel motions is 6 to 7 in 24 hours but can range from 1 to 20. The consistency of stool passed is usually thin, similar to the consistency of baby food. About 45% of patients have some form of dietary restriction. This means that they can eat any food they wish; however, some foods will cause them to have increased bowel motions and they will probably choose to avoid these. Ninety-seven percent reported no sexual limitations. One of the remarkable things that a pelvic pouch does is eliminate the sense of urgency experienced by most patients with UC. Urgency is the intense feeling of needing to get to a toilet right away or risk incontinence (loss of stool). Only 3% of patients after a pelvic pouch continue to routinely experience urgency. Of note, I usually tell patients that it takes about a year after they start to use their pelvic pouch before optimal pouch function is reached.

In an attempt to further improve the quality of these patients' lives after surgery, some may be placed on antidiarrheal medication such as a bulking agent (Metamucil, or Citrucel [SmithKline Beecham, Pittsburgh, PA]), Imodium (Janssen Pharmaceutica Inc., Titusville, NJ), or Lomotil (Searle and Co., Chicago, IL). Up to 47% of our patients sometimes take one of these medications.

Medical diagnosis is not an exact science. One point that needs mentioning is that even when we truly believe that the colonic dis-

ease is UC, there is a chance that it is Crohn's disease (CD). Sometimes even experienced gastroenterologists, surgeons, and pathologists find it very difficult to make the precise diagnosis. We found
7% of patients ultimately were found to have CD and in some this
was not diagnosed until 10 years after the pelvic pouch was constructed. This does not automatically mean the pelvic pouch must
be removed and in many patients the symptoms can be controlled
with medication. Symptoms may include pouch ulceration, urgency,
recurrent pouchitis, excessive bowel movements, anal abscesses,
and others.

A common problem seen in up to one third of patients after a
pelvic pouch is small bowel obstruction. This can result from kink-
ing related to adhesions or scar tissue. Of all patients experiencing
small bowel obstruction, about one third will require an operation to
release the adhesions.

As described for the continent ileostomy, patients with a pelvic
pouch may develop pouchitis. It will occur in up to one third of
patients and some will experience repeat attacks. Similar to symptoms for the continent ileostomy, patients with a pelvic pouch and
pouchitis may experience pelvic pressure or pain, increased bowel
movements, rectal bleeding, fevers, malaise, or joint aches. Some
have described an episode of pouchitis as a "miniattack of colitis."
In most circumstances it can be treated with medication such as
metronidazole. The cause of this problem is unknown.

When a pelvic pouch is constructed a temporary "loop" ileostomy
is frequently constructed to allow the numerous suture and staple
lines of the pouch to heal before stool passes through the pouch.
(This is a temporary stoma and managed in conjunction with specially trained nurses who teach patients to care for and cope with
having stomas enterostomal therapy [ET] nurses). The stoma may
need to be located in a less than ideal location so that it will reach
the surface of the abdomen and not pull on the pouch. The temporary stoma may be more difficult to pouch and have an increased
output. The increased output results from a moderate amount of
small bowel from the stoma to the anus that is not in circuit (stool
does not pass through it). This "out-of-circuit" bowel cannot come in
contact with feces to absorb fluid. I usually remind my patients that
this is a temporary problem and with diligent care from the ET

nurses and the use of antidiarrheal medication such as Lomotil or Imodium, the stoma can be managed successfully.

Anal skin is very sensitive and the stool that comes from the pelvic pouch can be irritating for some patients. Trying to decrease the frequency of bowel movements with antidiarrheal medications may be all that is needed but for some patients this is not enough. Many patients find that avoiding citrus fruits, chocolate, caffeine, spices, and/or fried foods can help. Direct protection of the anal skin with zinc oxide (e.g., Desitin baby ointment) (purchased from the grocery store or the pharmacy) is a mainstay of treatment. It provides a protective coating that is a barrier to the stool. I recommend liberal application and not attempting to completely wipe it off after defecation. Additionally, wiping with unscented baby wipes or moistened facial tissue can be gentler to the anal skin. Avoidance of dry toilet paper is recommended. If there is any stool leakage or seepage between bowel movements, placing a dry cotton ball by the anus to wick away moisture can be helpful. If the problem is severe, consult your doctor or ET nurse as other prescription medication may be needed.

One final thought before leaving the topic of pelvic pouches: The idea that because most patients have an acceptable outcome they no longer need to be followed by a doctor is *wrong*. We recommend a yearly pouch check along with biopsies to rule out any abnormality in the pelvic pouch. This exam is not as uncomfortable as previous endoscopies, such as the flexible sigmoidoscopy or colonoscopy, because there is only about 6 in. of pelvic pouch to examine. It usually does not require any sedation and at the Cleveland Clinic we do not even require any bowel preparation. (However, occasionally a patient will require an enema if the pouch is filled with stool.) Since the majority of patients with pelvic pouches receive them before the age of 30, they will live long lives with their pouch. We do not think there will be any problems with the pouch, but it is only through diligent follow-up that we can be sure. Additionally, if the pouch was constructed by the double-staple technique, a small rim of mucosa or lining tissue is left just above the anal control muscles. This 2-in. rim of tissue has the potential to have colon cells, and even though these cells may have some low-grade colitis and not cause any symptoms, it is important to biopsy this area to rule out any pre-cancerous changes.

CROHN'S DISEASE

CD is a more extensive problem than UC and can affect the intestinal tract anywhere from the mouth to the anus. The type of surgery and the functional outcome naturally depends on the section of bowel that requires operation. It is important to remember that CD is not "cured" by surgery. Surgery is planned when the symptoms are no longer manageable with medication or the complications of medication are not tolerable, or when the CD progresses to include infection, bleeding, obstruction of the bowel, or perforation (producing a hole in the bowel). Many patients wonder if their life span will be shortened from having CD. There have been no studies that have indicated that patients with CD live shorter lives than patients without the disease.

Small Intestine

A common site of CD is the distal small bowel where it enters the large intestine: the terminal ileum. Operation to remove this area of the bowel usually results in the ability to rejoin the end of the small intestine to the large intestine (anastomosis). There is a valve between the small and large bowel that is removed with an ileocolic resection. Bowel function after this type of surgery may not be changed. However, most patients usually report at least two bowel movements daily and some have four or more daily. If there is not CD in the colon, rectum, or anus, there usually is no problem with urgency or control of stool. The consistency of the stool may be loose from the amount of bowel removed or from the passage of bile salts directly into the large bowel instead of being absorbed in the distal small bowel. Usually, stool that is loose enough to cause significant symptoms can be managed with medication.

When operating for CD it is important to preserve as much small intestine as possible. In the past surgeons falsely believed that removing the abnormal small bowel with a large margin of normal bowel prevented the disease from returning or delayed the return of disease. Through studies it has been learned that this is incorrect. Currently, only significantly diseased bowel is removed. If there is a short segment of bowel that is affected by CD, an operation to enlarge the diameter of the bowel (strictureplasty) is performed. There can be multiple strictures in the small intestine from CD and in one patient at our institution more than 25 strictureplasties were done to preserve small intestine. This operation may be done in conjunction with resection of severely diseased bowel. Usually the overall bowel function is not affected.

The condition that this bowel preservation surgery is attempting to avoid is "short bowel syndrome." This is a rare consequence of extensive or multiple resections of small intestine. Patients afflicted typically cannot absorb enough calories to maintain their nutrition. They may need a special intravenous catheter that provides intravenous nutrition to survive. A commonly asked question after surgery is how much small bowel was removed. It is more important to ask your surgeon how much small bowel is remaining. The average person has 350 to 600 cm of small intestine. In general, loss of 50% to 70% of the small intestine can lead to problems. Additionally, patients with less than 100 cm of small intestines may have significant malabsorption and malnutrition.

Vitamin B_{12} is absorbed in the terminal ileum. The amount that can be resected without resulting in the inability to absorb the vitamin varies from person to person. If a significant portion of the terminal ileum has been removed, the blood level of B_{12} should be checked. We usually wait 3 to 6 months after surgery to check the blood level as this gives one's body the opportunity to use up any stores of the vitamin. Replacement is by monthly shots. Oral vitamin supplements will not replace this vitamin.

Kidney stones formed from calcium oxalate are more frequently seen in patients with CD who have had the terminal ileum removed. Actually the process involves oxalate (not calcium) entering the colon and being absorbed into the bloodstream. The concentration increases in the urine and binds to the calcium creating the stones. Diets that are low in oxalate are prescribed for patients with frequent attacks and problems with stones. Nutritional instruction with a dietitian is invaluable to help these patients.

Probably one of the most frequently asked questions centers around the risk of recurrence of CD after surgical resection. We have found 14 years after initial operation for patients with small bowel disease that 32% (±6%) required further surgery. For patients with

undergo surgery that entails creation of a stoma. This means bringing a section of intestine to the surface of the abdomen to eliminate bodily waste products. The underlying diseases vary including cancer, trauma, fecal incontinence (lack of control of stool), diverticulitis, and IBD. About one quarter of patients undergoing stoma construction have an ileostomy for IBD. For patients with colonic CD requiring surgery, the chance of needing a permanent ileostomy is very high. Adjustment reactions to permanent stomas vary as much as the individuals themselves. Concerns include odor, leakage, loss of sexual attractiveness, and loss of control of one's body. Also entering into a patient's adjustment is the family's perspective on the stoma. Modern ostomy equipment is odor-proof, flat under clothing, and comes in a variety of sizes and styles. Perhaps one of the most valuable assets is education provided by a trained expert. At my institution this entails an extensive preoperative visit from an ET nurse who has been trained to deal with the physical adaptation to the stoma and through extensive experience can pick up some of the emotional problems. Then we address these problems in a team approach with the patient. In some cases a consultation with a psychiatrist or psychologist is needed. Attempting to minimize ostomy appliance problems is one of the starting points and this entails marking a spot on the abdomen preoperatively that is on a flat surface and away from skin creases or bony prominence. Technically, construction of the stoma is crucial to decrease problems with appliance adherence. Then during the hospital recovery the ET nurse pays multiple visits to the patient in order to teach stoma care and provide emotional support. There are hundreds of products on the market used for stomal care. The product variation conforms with the differences in the contour of a patient's abdomen and the preferences he or she has for certain types of appliances. During the post operative course it is important for the ET nurse to examine the patient's goals and provide the type of appliance that is most suitable. Family education should also be included to dispel myths surrounding ostomies. Studies appear to show that patients with symptomatic colitis adjust better to a stoma than patients with cancer. Perhaps this is because removing a diseased colon due to IBD results in a significant improvement in overall health, whereas removing a cancer might not. The cancer may have caused minimal symptoms, and the patient may be preoccupied with the life-threatening prospect of recurrence of the cancer.

Another important area used to assist patients in coping with their stoma involves speaking to other patients who have a stoma. The United Ostomy Association is an organization committed to patients with stomas. They have support groups and new-patient visitation programs. These new-patient visits can be very helpful to the new ostomy patient. One suggestion to cope with problems centers around patients envisioning a "worst case scenario" to anticipate problems. Two examples cited by Margaret Goldberg, a noted ET nurse who also has a stoma, are as follows: Think what course of action you could take at a social gathering if your pouch leaked. One person pretended to spill coke on her clothes and was happy to have people perceive her as clumsy rather than incontinent. Another worst case scenario involved a patient in the middle of a college exam. Her stoma began to function loudly, so she feigned a coughing spell and excused herself to get a drink thus allowing her stoma to quiet down. Mentally planning ahead can help patients handle otherwise embarrassing situations.

One thing I try to stress to my patients is that a stoma does not mean the end of an active life. I have patients who are very active and not slowed a bit from their ileostomies. Notable examples include a man in his 50s who explores caves and is underground for up to 18 hours at a time. He had UC and preferred an ileostomy over a pelvic pouch secondary to his prolonged time underground. Another patient, a young woman, is a model who displays one-piece swim wear with her ileostomy. Several other women wear high-waisted two- piece swim suits to the beach. (Additionally, there are accessory ostomy products including pouch covers and fancy underclothing to enhance self-image.) I have had a high school student who played football and many patients who still enjoy swimming, horseback riding, skiing, snowmobiling, and other physical activities.

Sexual function is perhaps the area of greatest embarrassment and concern for patients. The alteration in body image can make them feel undesirable and repulsive. Sexual dysfunction from surgery for IBD in men is rare. Sexual desire is not usually physiologically affected but in rare cases nerves that trigger erection and ejaculation may be affected by surgery in the pelvis. This will require a thorough evaluation usually by a urologist who specializes in the treatment of these problems. Women usually worry about the ability to conceive and bear children. There have been no studies that have definitely shown that fertility is decreased in women after a stoma. In fact, the removal of the diseased colon may promote fertility. The enlarging uterus during pregnancy may necessitate a change in stoma appliances. But this problem can usually be remedied with the aid of an ET nurse. Table 1 gives recommendations for reducing anxiety about sexual activity in patients with ostomies.

Perianal Disease

Crohn's perianal disease encompasses a wide range of problems. They range from complex fistula (this is a tunnel connecting the

TABLE 1. *Recommendations for reducing anxiety about sexual activity in patients with ostomies*

1. Use good personal hygiene. Empty the pouch and seal before sexual activity.
2. Deodorize the pouch and avoid foods that cause gas, strong urinary odors, or loose stool 6 to 12 hours before sexual activity. In case the stoma "speaks out" (eliminates flatus), have a response rehearsed to minimize embarrassment.
3. If the ostomy is dry or controllable with irrigation, a minipouch that pops on and off an adhesive wafer is an option. Patients with ileostomies can also use this pouch. A flange cap that attaches to the adhesive wafer is also helpful. A drainable pouch may be tucked into a support belt, turned sideways, or taped down so that it will not flap in a distracting way.
4. Opaque pouch covers may be used to conceal fecal material. Other options include making a pouch cover to match other lingerie; covering with cummerbund, belt, or lightweight girdle; and wearing underwear with an opening up the center or satin boxer shorts. There is also lingerie/underwear made with pockets on the inside to hold the pouch.
5. To protect from leakage, a rubber sheet may be placed under the sheet, as well as a towel on top of the sheet. Remind the patient to keep a sense of humor should leakage occur, and plan to finish sexual activity in the bath or shower.
6. Experiment with sexual positions other than the missionary position, which may irritate or rub on the stoma.
7. Vaginal lubricants may be helpful to women with lubrication problems during arousal. Replens and Lubrin are both available over-the-counter and tend to be more suitable than K-Y jelly because they last longer.

Reprinted with permission from Shell JA. The psychosexual impact of ostomy surgery. *Progressions* 1992;4:14.

inside of the anus to the skin around the anus), abscesses around the anus, fissures (cracks in the anal lining), anal stenosis, and large external skin tags.

Most abscesses in the anal area should be drained both for comfort and to avoid extension of infection. Drainage catheters shaped like a mushroom are commonly used and left in place sometimes for an indefinite length of time. If a fistula develops, a flat drain that resembles a rubber band can be inserted. This drain is called a *seton* and also is left in place indefinitely. The most important principle is to drain the pus and prevent the ends from sealing, which would allow the process to begin again. Many patients wonder if they will be able to carry on all of their regular activities, including sexual intercourse, with such a drain. The device should not interfere with intercourse and will allow control of pain that results from buildup of fluid and pus.

In selected patients an operation can be done to close the inner lining of the fistula and eliminate the chronic drains and recurrent infection. This operation involves raising a flap of rectal lining tissue and covering the internal opening with this tissue. It is usually only about 50% to 60% successful in patients with CD.

Anal fissures from CD are often located in the lateral (3 o'clock or 9 o'clock) position. They usually are asymptomatic, so that any pain should be evaluated for infection. For fissures that are symptomatic secondary to spasm from exposed anal muscle (exposed due to the crack in the lining over the muscle), a limited division of this spasming muscle as would be done for a non-Crohn's fissure can be done. This risks the occurrence of a nonhealing wound or possible problems with the ability to control stool. Medical treatment may be the best option and should include metronidazole and/or steroid suppositories.

Mild anal stenosis (narrowing of the anal opening) is usually well tolerated. Anal dilatation is usually done cautiously as it may result in incontinence.

Many patients have large tags of skin at their anus and misinterpret them as hemorrhoids. Usually no surgery is done for these tags as the wounds tend to heal poorly.

Some patients with perianal CD exhibit no disease elsewhere in the intestinal tract. Nonetheless, if the anal disease is complicated or severe enough, only a stoma to divert the fecal stream away from the anus will alleviate the symptoms.

CONCLUSION

Life goes on after surgery for IBD. The most important point from the patient's perspective is to ask questions and obtain as much information as possible about the procedure. If a stoma may be necessary, assistance from an ET nurse both before and after surgery is crucial. Also, support groups such as those sponsored by the Crohn's and Colitis Foundation of America, the United Ostomy Association, or your local hospital are beneficial in aiding the adjustment to life after surgery.

SUGGESTED READINGS

Croushore EE, Steiger E. Short bowel syndrome. In: Fazio VW, ed. *Current therapy in colon and rectal surgery.* Philadelphia: B.C. Decker, 1990;347–354.

Fazio VW. Crohn's disease of the small bowel. In: Fazio VW, ed. *Current therapy in colon and rectal surgery.* Philadelphia: BC Decker, 1990;358–363.

Fazio VW, Ziv Y, Church JM, Oakley JR, Lavery IC, Milsom JW, Schroeder TK. The ileal pouch-anal anastomoses: complications and function in 1005 patients. *Ann Surg* 1995;222:120–127.

Goldberg MT. Promoting positive self-concept in patients with stomas: nursing interventions. *Progressions* 1991;3:3–12.

Hull TL, Erwin-Toth P. The pelvic pouch procedure and continent ostomies: overview and controversies. *J Wound Ostomy Continence Nurs* 1996;23:156–165.

Kock NG. Intra-abdominal "reservoir" in patients with permanent ileostomy. Preliminary observations on a procedure resulting in fecal continence in five ileostomy patients. *Arch Surg* 1969;99:223–231.

Mueller V. Quality of life after ostomy: individualizing assessment and care. *Progressions* 1993;5:3–15.

Parks AG, Nicholls RJ. Proctocolectomy without ileostomy for ulcerative colitis. *Br Med J* 1978;2:85–88.

Shell JA. The psychosexual impact of ostomy surgery. *Progressions* 1992;4:3–15.

Walsh BA, Grunert BK, Telford GL, Otterson MF. Multidisciplinary management of altered body image in the patient with an ostomy. *J Wound Ostomy Continence Nurs* 1995;22:227–236.

CHAPTER 13

ALTERNATIVE MEDICINE

Samuel D. Benjamin

GENERAL PERSPECTIVE

While there is continued progress in the treatment of inflammatory bowel disease (IBD), more and more individuals are turning to
alternative modalities as possible methods of relieving symptoms in
those afflicted with IBD. Perhaps the biggest single problem is that
there is no responsible and scientifically based fountain of information with regard to what is safe in alternative therapies, what the
potential effect of the alternative therapy is, and what the long-term
effects of using alternative modalities are. Many traditional medicine
texts regard alternative providers as "quacks." Other texts in book
stores purporting the advantage of alternative modalities suggest that
allopathic, or Western, medicine is of no utility and that it is merely
a way of decreasing one's own defenses by the use of immunosup-

University Center for Complementary and Alternative Medicine at Stony Brook,
State University of New York at Stony Brook Health Sciences Center, Stony
Brook, New York 11794

pressants and thereby endangering one in the long run—a conspiracy of the uncaring medical establishment.

In fact, there is increasing evidence that alternative modalities are being used throughout the United States in record numbers. A study done by David Eisenberg at Harvard Medical School and Beth Israel Hospital in 1990 was published in *New England Journal of Medicine* in 1993. That study showed that nearly one-third of all Americans had used alternative therapies the year before. Interestingly, this study did not include children below the age of 18, and it did not include people who, because of their ethnic background, did not speak English well enough to assure the telephone surveyor that the information received was accurate. Therefore, it is not unreasonable to assume that alternative therapies may indeed be used by an even larger percentage of the population.

Of particular note is the increasingly positive response of the established medical community, of corporate America, and of insurance companies throughout the United States to develop safe programs in integrative medicine. Throughout the rest of this discussion, I will use the term "integrative medicine" to refer to the integration of allopathic medicine and alternative therapies, giving you what I believe to be the most options for the treatment of IBD.

From the outset, it is important to acknowledge the incredible value of allopathic medicine. I would be wary of any physician or practitioner who suggests that you should not be treated with Western medical care or does not want to coordinate their activities with your gastroenterologist or primary care physician (PCP). Undoubtedly, the "state of the art" in the treatment of IBD both in general and specifically is to be sure that there is a close working relationship between the alternative medicine physician/provider and the gastroenterologist/PCP.

The choice of gastroenterologist is very important. The physician must be willing to work with you in the utilization of alternative therapies. There are increasing numbers of gastroenterologists throughout the United States who are developing skills in integrative medicine. If you are interested in exploring integrative treatments and the gastroenterologist feels that it is inappropriate, then I would recommend that you first consider the rationale of your gastroenterologist. Should you still feel that you wish to use an integrative approach, you should seek out providers who are willing to work with you as you explore other options for your care.

Equally, it is key that you choose providers in alternative therapies who can offer you safe options and who are willing to work with your gastroenterologist. Unfortunately, in the United States at the present time, there is barely any appropriate credentialing of providers in alternative medicine. In New York State and in a number of states throughout the United States, there is a requirement that physicians and nonphysician acupuncturists complete minimum standards before they can practice. However, in many states physicians and nonphysicians can treat people with acupuncture, homeopathy, herbal medicine, massage, and the like without licensure or minimum requirements. In addition, the language of alternative medicine is oftentimes quite different than that of Western medicine. Terminology and the way health is addressed are different. You must seek out providers who can and will communicate with each other. Alternative treatments must not effect your Western treatment adversely.

It is not unreasonable to say that many nonphysician healers offer options worth exploring. However, there is a shortfall that must be carefully considered. That is, the nonphysician does not have the complete breadth and understanding of the medical problem from a Western perspective. I think it is this kind of global knowledge that makes the practitioner more effective in the integration of medical services. Therefore, I would more strongly recommend that you seek the care of a physician or a physician group that coordinates activities in alternative medicine with allopathic care.

Individuals with Crohn's disease (CD) can oftentimes, because of chronic antibiotic administration and steroid use, be more susceptible to infection. The appropriate choice becomes quite important when performing a sterile technique such as acupuncture. While extraordinarily uncommon, the acupuncture needle could theoretically perforate the peritoneum and cause an infection. This is incredibly rare in the hands of skilled practitioners who follow careful medical hygiene and technique. However, there is no protection for the individual when in the hands of an unlicensed practitioner whose training may come from either a few short weeks of attendance in a course or, for that matter, from a correspondence course. In addition, it is important to identify when someone is having an acute episode that may not be appropriate for alternative modality therapy.

Lastly, as stated at the beginning of this discussion, it is really important for you to recognize how important it is not to give up standard medical treatments when beginning alternative therapies. Some of the comments that are made by some alternative practitioners include:

1. "We need to cleanse your body of the toxins from standard medical care."
2. "We need to free your body of all present treatments in order for our treatment to work." Or,
3. "It is impossible to have a mind, body, and spiritual healing as long as you are on these medications."

These are red flags that should make you very wary of the provider. I would not work with anyone who espouses this kind of approach.

I think it is realistic to look to healing rather than to cure. I do not know of any substantive data at the present time relative to alternative modalities that "cure" IBD. However, I think that there is an increasing body of experience that suggests alternative modalities can substantially decrease the suffering and complications associated with IBD on their own or when coupled with standard allopathic care.

I do not want to sound negative about alternative medicine, but I think that we need to be sure we have a realistic perspective with regard to alternative modalities. You need to be sure that you are using a provider who is well trained and has a good understanding of when to use alternative medicine, when to use allopathic care, and how to combine them. You need to be sure their credentials are appropriate. In addition, you need to know if your insurance company does or does not cover alternative therapies.

INSURANCE COVERAGE IN ALTERNATIVE MEDICINE FOR INFLAMMATORY BOWEL DISEASE

There are still relatively few insurance companies, either in managed care or in the standard indemnity insurance, that cover integrative medicine. These are, however, increasing at a rapid rate. The reason for this is because as one insurance company in your area offers integrative medicine coverage, so will all the other companies in the area in order to avoid losing part of their "market share." This is an important tool for you because insurance companies are now very sensitive to market demand.

If you or your employer are favorably disposed to integrative medicine, then you need to clearly express this to your insurer who will respond by seeking out the appropriate network of alternative medicine providers who also meet the Western medical qualifications of the National Council for Quality Assurance (NCQA). In the United States, managed care insurance companies have taken the lead in promoting integrative medicine. The reason is that the managed care insurance companies are evolving to provide choice and quality. In the future, managed care insurance companies will survive only if they decrease cost, improve the quality of care, and respond to the needs of their patients (insureds).

MEDICAL TRAINING

Allopathic medical schools, i.e., medical schools that confer the degree of medical doctor (M.D.), are increasingly aware of the need to train their medical students in alternative medicine. At present, there are approximately 52 undergraduate training programs in medical schools throughout the United States, and this number is increasing every year. Osteopathic medical schools that teach osteopathic manipulation are also including other areas of integrative medicine such as herbal medicine and homeopathy in their undergraduate curriculum. Osteopathic medical colleges confer the degree of doctor of osteopathy (D.O.).

Many allopathic teaching institutions are also developing residency training programs that include integrative medicine. A residency training program is a postgraduate program that either an allopathic or osteopathic physician trains in for a varying period of time in order to receive specialty credentials in family practice, internal medicine, obstetrics/gynecology, pediatrics, etc. There is such a program in integrative medicine at the Hennepin County Hospital in Minneapolis, Minnesota. At the State University of New York at Stony Brook we are planning a residency training program that will include an extra year of integrative medicine. A number of other residency training programs in integrative medicine that will include a specialty in primary health care with particular emphasis on integrative medical services are being planned throughout the United States.

At the time of writing, two fellowship programs are already up and running in integrative medicine. A fellowship program is a 1- to 2- year training program in a specialized area that an allopathic or osteopathic physician can take once they have completed their specialty or residency training. At the University of Maryland and the University of Arizona, fellowships are available in integrative medicine and the National Institutes of Health has a research fellowship available as well.

There are many institutions that train acupuncturists, herbalists, energy medicine specialists, lay homeopaths, and so forth. I strongly recommend that your first encounter in integrative medicine be coordinated by a licensed physician or nurse practitioner well versed in integrative medicine who can help you interact with these individuals.

At your first consultation in integrative medicine, it is important that you bring all of your past medical history, lab tests, diagnostic testing, and herbs or homeopathic remedies that you may have tried on your own. Ideally, as in any consultation, it is useful to get this information to the provider as early as possible. If you have not seen an allopathic provider in a long time, then a traditional examination done by the integrative physician or a member of his or her staff is vital. You should come prepared to answer some very detailed and often intimate questions with regard to yourself and your family. Questions such as how things are going at home, what your favorite color is, and what your favorite season is may be asked. The integrative physician is interested in securing detailed information about your home, workplace, family, family history, medical history, sexual history, environmental history, and dietary history to name but a few. Some of the questions might seem nonsensical and this should not disturb you. Alternative modalities of treatment and diagnoses are based on very different concepts and often are very different approaches from allopathic medicine. Often what appears to be a nonlinear way of thinking does indeed have a point. It is not unreasonable to parallel alternative medicine to allopathic medicine as one would compare chaos mathematics to basic arithmetic. Both are valid philosophies and both are complementary. The doctor is looking for very subtle, nearly inconsequential signs and symptoms in order to facilitate your treatment.

The physical examination might include merely holding you, putting hands over you, feeling pulses in both wrists, looking at your tongue and perhaps the palms of your hands, as well as observing the architecture of your ears. This is Traditional Chinese Medicine. The provider might talk about *chakras*. This is Aryuvdeic medicine practiced by tens of thousands of healers in India with a history of some 5,000 years. These terms hopefully will not incite doubt or fear but instead should trigger your curiosity.

Do these technologies with their strange terminology suggest that healing can be done "magically?" I think it better to consider terms like *qi* (pronounced *chi*), the life source in traditional Chinese medicine, as allegorical descriptions for scientific concepts that we have yet to grasp. I often use these terms in my office for want of a more westernized expression to describe the same concept.

Very often, the integrative medical office will provide, either through your insurance company or upon your direct purchase, herbal products and homeopathic remedies. I think that while I believe there can be implicit problems with conflict of interest (namely, that profits increase when a health care provider sells these products), there is also some benefit in that a good integrative physician has taken the time to explore the kinds and brands of herbal and homeopathic products that he or she is handling and has attempted to secure the best quality.

Just as you would in any other physician's office, it is important that you gaze about to be sure things are clean, e.g., that acupuncture needles are appropriately stored either in sterilized containers or in presterilized disposable packets. It is important that the pillows and sheets be changed after each patient and that you ask if the examination tables are cleaned down with Cidex to ensure that there is no spread of infection from one patient to the other. This would be no different from what you would expect in any doctor's office, so trust your intuition! If the office does not look clean, then you should not be there! Just because one of your friends tells you that this physician worked a "miracle" is not evidence enough. If the provider makes you feel uncomfortable you should leave. If the provider sounds loving and committed, that's great! Someone who sounds like a charlatan probably is! This is sound advice whether it is a physician in alternative medicine or a physician engaged in allopathic practice. An integrative physician should be warm, friendly, non-confrontational, and should spend a considerable amount of time with you on the first visit. He or she should be working toward empowering you to deal with this problem, not just "plugging in" a new kind of technology whether it be acupuncture, homeopathy, or herbal medicine as if it were just another form of allopathic treatment. Integration means uniting the mind, body, and spirit. It means addressing not just the individual but the family and community. Beware of a physician who wants to "cure" you with any single method such as acupuncture. Integrative medicine is a coordinated approach.

TREATMENT MODALITIES

Introduction

Generally speaking, there has been very little clinical research in the alternative methodologies used to treat IBD. Much of what I am about to discuss is based on empirical information only. There is an enormous need for more detailed scientific studies to address what is efficacious in alternative therapy for the treatment of IBD. The problem has been that much of the conventional medical community, including medical teaching institutions, have looked askance at alternative therapies and have disregarded most of it as being "unscientific" and therefore ineffective. In fact, this notion is unfortunate because without looking at whether or not these modalities make a difference, we cannot realistically support or criticize the use of any treatment modality.

The problem is that if you or a family member is suffering from IBD and the traditional medical model of treatment is not entirely successful, or if you are concerned about long-term side effects, we should not necessarily discourage you from using any of the following treatment modalities provided that they do not interfere with your present therapy and that they *do no harm.*

Herbal Remedies

Aloe vera

The aloe vera plant, indigenous to hot climates, is effective in the treatment of IBD as a juice. I prefer to use 99% pure aloe vera juice that is not from a concentrate and uses the whole aloe vera plant. Oftentimes it is cheaper to purchase aloe vera concentrate, but in my opinion this is far less effective. It is also important to remember dosages. One to three teaspoons 3 times a day is more than effective in an adult and the pediatric dose should be about one-half to one-fourth of that amount. While you can certainly experiment with higher doses, my greatest concern is the potential for diarrhea as the dose increases. Aloe vera juice is receiving some attention in the conventional medical literature as a potential therapy to both treat chronic recurrent cases and decrease the recrudescence rate of IBD, i.e., CD and ulcerative colitis.

Slippery elm bark

Slippery elm bark is helpful for treatment of both acute and chronic cases of IBD. I do not know of any reported cases of drug interaction between steroids, immunosuppressants, and/or antiinflammatory drugs and the slippery elm bark, so I would feel comfortable using it concomitantly with conventional therapy. Slippery elm bark can be taken either in a gruel form or in a freeze-dried form found typically in many health food stores; I find the latter to be much more convenient. Slippery elm in freeze-dried form comes in pills. For adults, the full dose varies but is usually approximately 740 mg of a standard extract 3 times a day taken either before, during, or after meals. Usually about half of the adult dosage is appropriate for children.

Chamomile

Chamomile can be taken either in a glycerin base, as a liquid, as a tincture, in freeze-dried form, or in a tea. Chamomile decreases the amount of intestinal spasm and should be taken only with the approval of the physician treating you for IBD. In addition, chamomile has a pleasant taste and a mild tranquilizing effect that is not habit forming and can be quite useful for the anxiety associated with IBD. Chamomile is not addictive.

Peppermint in enteric-coated capsules

Peppermint acts as an antispasmodic. It is safe and effective and does not have some of the more troublesome effects of crossing the blood–brain barrier such as commercial products like Bentyl or Levsin. The trick is to be sure that the peppermint is in an oil within

an enteric-coated capsule because if released in the stomach (susceptible to gastric acids), the antispasmodic effect of the peppermint is
substantially decreased. *Warning:* peppermint will increase gastroe-
sophageal reflux disease if you suffer from this as well. In past years,
people would take peppermint after a meal in order to burp, thought to
be a sign of good digestion. This can be a problem if you are taking
drugs that are irritating to the lining of the esophagus such as steroid
products or nonsteroidal antiinflammatory drugs causing "heartburn."

PHYSICAL MEDICINE

Manipulation therapy

From the outset, I think that both osteopathic manipulation and chiropractic care can offer improvement for the symptoms of IBD. Once
again, there is a sparsity of studies to support this and what I am pre-
senting here is based on observation. I do feel that gentle manipulation
done by an experienced practitioner can do no harm. The issue here is
to be sure that this is *gentle manipulation.* I, for one, prefer manipulation in the cranial field although certainly other practitioners have
proven other areas of manipulation to be effective with many of my
patients. I do not believe that "back cracking," as we often expect of
people who do manipulative care, is necessary to get an efficacious
treatment. At the time of preparing this chapter, I believe that there are
only about 300 board-certified osteopathic manipulative physicians in
the United States. There are numerous schools of chiropractic treatment with varying standards, and I think it is important to ask your
physical medicine provider about his or her professional background
and training. Most chiropractors are responsible practitioners; however, some speak out against immunizations and much of allopathic
medicine. Beware of these extremists. Find someone who is willing to
integrate, not isolate. Osteopaths are in all states of the United States
allowed to prescribe conventional medicine.

Massage therapy

There are many different forms that massage therapy can take and
my strongest advice is to look for massage therapy that makes you feel
comfortable. Massages that are so vigorous as to cause pain or nausea

have not been shown to be more effective in helping with some of the symptoms and the anxiety associated with IBD than less aggressive techniques and should never be administered! There are many forms of massage therapy including polarity, Swedish massage, therapeutic massage, and so forth. I think it is best to experiment a bit with what makes you feel comfortable. In our health centers we have had considerable success combining manipulation in the cranial field with massage therapy. Patients seem to have fewer complaints about flare-ups or abdominal pain. I do not think that we have been able to correlate a direct relationship between the use of physical medicine and decreasing the amount of blood or mucus in the stools, for example. Once again, I do not see any contraindication to the use of manipulative and physical medicine along side conventional therapies.

Before ending this section, let us touch on methodologies such as tai chi and yoga. No physician would argue the importance of keeping one's body flexible and in good shape. This is especially important in patients who use steroid products that can cause osteoporosis and make their bones more susceptible to trauma. Therefore balance and flexibility seem to me to be paramount in the treatment of a patient with IBD. Both tai chi and yoga offer many different ways of dealing with these issues. I do not think we need to become fanatical in our pursuit of these disciplines. One does not have to pursue them as a religion. They can be taught without challenging your personal beliefs. I would also suggest that you look for an instructor who recognizes that you may be more susceptible to stress fractures than the average person before you begin exercising so that he or she can design a program that best fits your needs.

Acupuncture and Traditional Chinese Medicine

While oftentimes in public we consider acupuncture to be a single entity, and in fact in many states it is licensed independently, acupuncture is a part of Traditional Chinese Medicine which includes many traditional Chinese herbal formulas. I believe that acupuncture itself can be very effective either independent of conventional medicine or jointly with conventional or allopathic treatments to address issues pertaining to IBD. Certainly, acupuncture can be very helpful in pain management associated with IBD. Acupuncture, however, is much less effective when the individual is on steroid medications. Therefore, I usually recommend that you do not cease steroid treatment but rather wait until you have been taken off steroids to begin acupuncture. If you are in an acute stage and there is little hope of tapering off steroids, then certainly trying acupuncture concomitantly is not unreasonable but one's expectations should be significantly lowered as to the efficacy of acupuncture in this situation. In short, I think that acupuncture is not only a pain management technique but should be an integral part of the standard treatment for IBD.

Traditional Chinese medical herbal combinations must be treated with a great deal of respect. As a rule, I advise my patients against their use. There is no question that there are numerous combinations that, in my opinion, can make significant differences in the course of IBD. It should be noted that the U.S. Food and Drug Administration (FDA) does not recognize most herbal treatments as accepted medical therapy. Therefore, the control in the production of herbal products is substantially less than one would expect of ethical pharmaceutical products. Many herbal products, including many that come from China, are contaminated with bacteria, protozoa, or chemical products that could be potentially harmful to an individual. Reports of kidney failure from Chinese herbs are increasing in the medical literature. Therefore, choosing a practitioner who knows the source of these products is very important. The FDA requires an investigational new drug application and research program to be prepared for each new pharmaceutical or pharmaceutical combination. The cost of such research can exceed $30 million before final approval is completed. This becomes an economically limiting factor for a pharmaceutical company because natural products utilized cannot be patented; therefore it would be hard to recap research expenses. While there has been some legislation to decrease some of the potential hazards of taking herbal products in the United States, by and large consumers must be very aware of what they are taking and why they are taking it to be sure they do not, in fact, exacerbate an attack of IBD. At present, most herbs are classified as food products and their production and marketing is poorly monitored and controlled by state and federal agencies.

An experienced herbalist or, even better, an experienced physician who is either treating you with alternative therapy or supervising an alternative therapist would at this point be your best protection against using herbal products that could potentially cause harm. One must remember that in traditional Chinese medicine as well as in acupuncture in general, the treatment is not directed to the disease—in this case IBD—but instead to treatment of a constellation of signs and symptoms that are expressed sometimes in very colorful terms such as "fire in the liver." While an alternative provider can see five different patients in a day with the same allopathic diagnosis of IBD, the treatment would vary from individual to individual because of the differences in their signs and symptoms. Traditional Chinese medicine does not "know" the diagnosis of IBD. A traditional Chinese physician might, for example, be treating the large intestine on one hand but also treating the kidney, which is the source of *qi* on the other hand. There is a wonderful book that I recommend for those who have some interest in this regard called *The Web That Has No Weaver*, written by Ted J. Kaptchuk, O.M.D. (Oriental Medical Doctor) which I think aptly explains Traditional Chinese Medicine.

Music and music beds

I have experimented with the use of a Therasound music bed. There are many different vehicles for using various frequencies to address corresponding frequencies in the human body. There is very little proof at this point that these treatments make any difference. I can tell you that I have yet to see them have any contraindication in the use of IBD and they do help to a certain amount in making the patient more at ease. Whether this is related in fact to the music and its frequency specifically or to a general feeling of well being that musical elicits in many of us, I cannot say. There is a great deal of research that is ongoing on the use of music as an integral part of treatment not just because it is soothing but, in fact, by having a direct influence on organ systems. I think it is sufficient to say that there really is no contraindication unless you have heart disease or a seizure disorder in which case we must be sure that the frequencies and volume being used in the treatment are not such that they would induce an untoward event.

Homeopathy

Homeopathy is perhaps the most controversial area of alternative medicine because at first blush its basic principle seems to be quite preposterous. Homeopathy is based on the law of similars, which suggests that the use of imperceptible or nearly imperceptible amounts of natural substances that can cause similar symptoms to the ones the patient exhibits can summon a natural healing response. Therefore, if one were to have a constellation of symptoms that include abdominal pain and diarrhea, then treating the individual with arsenic that had been diluted to the point where there is only one molecule of arsenic in the solution or pill being given, or no perceptible amount of arsenic identified in that solution, will elicit a healing response in the body that will stop the diarrhea. In other words, like treats like. Something that can cause diarrhea when diluted greatly can eliminate diarrhea. To get even more complex, however, in that it is not just treating diarrhea but in fact there are many different remedies to treat diarrhea depending on many other circumstances. For example, are there accompanying problems with the stools? Does the individual have one of multiple different personalities that can be described? In fact, the problem is that homeopathic medicine in some ways is like the dilemma of finding a needle in a haystack, i.e., a very complex set of symptoms that must be precisely matched with a homeopathic remedy.

From the point of view of traditional modern medicine, this does not seem to have any logical basis. How could something that causes the symptoms in fact treat the symptoms? Further, how could something that has a barely perceptible dose or no perceptible dose cure a "real" disease? Certainly there are already precedents within standard allopathic medicine. Allergy shots, or desensitization, is in fact a homeopathic treatment in that small doses of something to which the individual is allergic are injected beneath the skin in an attempt to cause the body to react less forcefully to the substance. So if one has ragweed sensitivity, then by injecting various tiny dilutions of ragweed underneath the skin the body could become "accustomed" to ragweed biologically and the allergy symptoms would decrease substantially. There are, in fact, some intriguing studies reported by the University of Glasgow School of Medicine treating children in pediatrics that must cause us to consider homeopathy as a potential and viable treatment for IBD.

Some of the advantages of homeopathy are that it is remarkably cheap, with treatments costing no more than $5 or $10 for several months, and that there are no real side effects that we cannot quantify at the present time from the individuals being thus treated. The danger would be in seeking homeopathic treatment before conventional care where conventional care could make a significant difference. I like to refer patients to physician homeopaths either for concomitant therapy or for homeopathic therapy only when their symptoms have totally subsided and if they are no longer using any standard conventional medicine. I would not use a homeopathic remedy in lieu of conventional medicine in an acute flare-up but would do so in a manner complimentary to allopathic treatment. Much research is needed to evaluate the validity of homeopathy.

Aromatherapy

I will mention aromatherapy only briefly. Clearly there are olfactory triggers in the limbic system of the brain as a result of certain kinds of odors. These odors may not even be perceived! One of the calming ones for intestinal or abdominal problems could be cedar and sandalwood. There are other possibilities depending on the individual. I have no objection to experimenting with aromatherapy as long as one recognizes that he or she might be allergic to some of the products causing the aroma. Aromatherapy can act both to calm moments of anxiety associated with IBD and to potentially offer some assistance in decreasing some of the pain and spasm of these kinds of therapies.

Mind/body (psychoneuroimmunology)

I will leave the question of whether IBD is an infectious or autoimmune disease or whether there are other genetic predispositions to my colleagues who specialize in this area. However, few if any of us can deny the importance of attitude in terms of healing. There are, at this point, numerous studies in literature not just specific to IBD but to many disease states and in particular with autoimmunity suggesting that the appropriate attitude, less fear, etc., makes a significant difference in the outcome of disease. A clear connection has been demonstrated between our attitude and chemicals in our brain and the rest of our body, called *neuropeptides*. In addition, our immune systems have allies producing messengers in many different organs—even from our red blood cells. They can, in fact, modulate our immune system, our blood pressure, our heart rate, etc. There are new techniques that are being used throughout the United States and that I have been using in my office to help individuals modulate the course of their disease. These techniques include guided visual imaging, mindfulness, meditation, biofeedback, and hypnosis—all ways of altering one's state of consciousness and attempting to "assist the body" in healing itself. These techniques have little if any side effect other than perhaps the anxiety of hoping that they work, and they offer a wonderful method for individuals to achieve self-empowerment. I like to use mind–body medicine to manage the pain of IBD as well as the actual course of IBD in flare-ups. Mind–body techniques can be used both in the acute stage as well as chronic stage of IBD and can be used concomitantly with any of the aforementioned therapies including conventional medicine. In fact, I would have to say at this point that it is mandatory that any patient with IBD be exposed to at least one if not several forms of mind–body technologies as a means of helping to control their disease. They can, in effect, tell the body to cool down their symptoms. There is an excellent document that reviews this approach by *Consumer Reports* entitled "Mind/Body Medicine" edited by Daniel Coleman and Joel Gurin that is readily available from Consumer Reports Publishers that I think offers a balanced approach to looking at this area and can be very useful for you in the selection of the specific form or technique that you would like to use. I would encourage you to ask the advice of your physician with regard to certified practitioners of visual imaging, mindfulness, or biofeedback in the community. Many physicians are certified in hypnotherapy. In addition, you can be trained in doing self-hypnosis, which is equally effective. Is there a difference between one form of mind/body medicine and another? Are there studies that show us when one may be more effective than another? I think at this point the jury is still out. Suffice it to say I do not think you can do any harm by utilizing these techniques, not only from the point of view of treating the illness directly but also because it will give you a true feeling of control and self-confidence.

I think it is particularly important to add that more studies are being done in group healing. There seems to be a clear pattern that people do better when they are in groups helping each other, supporting each other, even holding each other. An excellent study by Dr. David Spiegel of Stanford University Medical School showed that women in caring groups lived longer with breast cancer than those who were in comparable groups. My clinical experience has shown that people show marked attitudinal changes and seem to fare better clinically by being in groups where the members tend to support each other. I want to point out that these are not the kinds of groups where individuals are lectured to by physicians or specialists in IBD, or where people "cry on each other's shoulders." These are groups whose members share a gamut of feelings including happiness and sadness, where they pray and meditate together, and where they share their real feelings and support each other. They may share massages together. They may do yoga or tai chi together. I am absolutely convinced of the benefits of groups and once again I see little danger in working in a group environment. I see no danger in using this kind of technique while taking conventional medicine at the present time.

Prayer

I have left prayer for the very last because for me there is no more powerful tool in healing. While this may sound like merely a noble statement from a committed individual, please make no mistake about it: Prayer is now undergoing a considerable amount of scientific investigation and the initial results are quite intriguing! In one study, a decreased length of stay in the hospital was demonstrated as a result of others praying for individuals even though they did not know it. There are numerous studies showing that when individuals pray, not necessarily for themselves but for others as well, they themselves seem to heal at a faster rate. From the outset I must admit to you my absolute faith and belief in God. I cannot tell you who practices the right religion. I cannot advise you in which way you should pray because we all pray in our own way. Some of you reading this may not necessarily belong to an organized religion but do believe in our interconnectedness and are spiritual people. In a number of studies that have been published recently, it is clear that physicians pray for their patients in ever increasing numbers. I (if permitted) pray with my patient at the time of the visit. I often find myself praying for my patients while riding home in my car or coming to work. We have patient groups that in effect are prayer chains for patients. These are patients who come from various walks of life, from diverse social, economic, and ethnic groups, and from different religions. In addition, many of our patients do not subscribe to any particular religion but do support the concept of a global spirituality. I cannot tell you if prayer is some unique force that we have not been able to adequately describe in the universe as of yet. As a scientist I am not supposed to subscribe to "magical" or "mystical" powers. For me it makes no difference whether I am a physician or a scientist; I am an individual as you are and we share a common heritage. Prayer, both from the point of view of our own humanity as well as from the point of view of science, should play a very important part in how you treat yourself and others with IBD. I have often heard of individuals who have been harmed by conventional medical therapies. I have yet to hear of a patient who has passed away from an overdose of prayer. There is one caveat, however: I do not believe in faith healing. Prayer is a complement to conventional and alternative therapies—not a standalone!

God gave us prayer *and* technology. We should use them together.

SUMMARY

In summary, there are a number of different techniques used to treat IBD that can be classified as alternative modalities. I believe that the best approach is to seek integrative medical care that combines conventional medical wisdom with alternative modalities in an environment that can do no harm and that is well controlled. Any individual with IBD who chooses this course of therapy must recognize that at the present time there are few data to support the efficacy of these kinds of treatments and that is why it is so important that they seek care from physicians who practice integrative medicine or physician groups that include alternative practitioners in a controlled environment. Herbal medicine, homeopathic medicine, physical medicine, and so forth are viable options that are available to patients and will give them an opportunity to enjoy self-empowerment and some independence from the present medical system, which often usurps the patient's ability to take control of his or her life and be autonomous. The most important point to remember is that it does not have to be an either/or process, that there are in fact physicians and physician groups available that will allow individuals to "experiment" with modalities in a safe and nurturing environment and permit them to enjoy more control over their healing process and over their lives.

CHAPTER 14

MAKING A DIFFERENCE: THE ROLE OF CCFA AND ITS SUPPORT OF PATIENTS

Lisa H. Richardson, Jane W. Present, and Marjorie Merrick

CCFA's mission is to raise funds:

To support basic and clinical scientific research to find the cause of, and cure for, Crohn's disease and ulcerative colitis;

To provide educational programs for patients, medical professionals, and the general public; and

To offer supportive services for patients, their families, and their friends.

CCFA's founders: Irwin M. Rosenthal, William D. Modell, and Henry D. Janowitz

Crohn's and Colitis Foundation of America Inc., New York, New York 10016

CCFA'S PROFILE

"Every year, approximately 30,000 Americans learn that they suffer from Crohn's Disease or ulcerative colitis."

The year 1997 marked the thirtieth anniversary of the Crohn's and Colitis Foundation of America (CCFA) as the only national voluntary, nonprofit organization in the United States devoted to IBD research, education, and supportive services for the estimated 2 million Americans affected by Crohn's disease (CD) and ulcerative colitis (UC). Supported solely by individuals, foundations, and corporate contributions, the CCFA (formally known as the National Foundation for Ileitis and Colitis, or NFIC) credits its success to the generosity, hard work, and dedication of so many individuals. The dynamic partnership between the lay and medical leaders developed in earlier years continues today stronger than ever. Over the years the third essential element of this mutually respectful alliance has been added, i.e., the Foundation's professional staff. A strong bond with the health care industry and government interacts with this partnership trio.

Today CCFA has 55 chapters, some of which have paid staff, and others that exist through the good will and commitment of loyal volunteers throughout the country. More than 150,000 members, donors, and friends have responded to its appeals for support and over 2,000 physicians, nurses, and health care professionals have become medical members.

With the national office located in New York City, CCFA consists of a board of trustees represented by its chapters all across the United States, and an executive committee of officers and specially appointed trustees who monitor all activities of the foundation and report to the board.

We have come a very long way since CCFA's founding in 1967. The foundation has experienced substantial financial growth through its fund raising and development efforts. As a result, CCFA has been able to increase education to individuals and families affected by IBD with services that have expanded from updated books and brochures to educational programs, support groups, videos, and an on-line computer system. Nearly $0.82 of every dollar raised is allocated to research and program services. The Better

Business Bureau and the National Charities Information Board (NCIB), which monitors not-for-profit agencies, have listed CCFA as one of the most fiscally responsible agencies in the country. Most importantly, CCFA now holds and/or has a presence in more medical workshops, educational symposia, and health-related conventions in any given year than we had during the first 25 years.

CCFA sponsored one national workshop in its first 20 years, bringing together scientists to discuss IBD research. Today the organization sponsors one workshop every 18 months and is represented at three national conventions each year sponsored by the American Gastroenterology Association, the American College of Gastroenterology, and the North American Society for Pediatric Gastroenterology and Nutrition.

SUPPORTING AND MAINTAINING
RESEARCH

"Since its creation in 1967, CCFA has awarded more than $44 million to researchers attempting to find the cause of and cure for CD and UC."

The National Scientific Advisory Committee (NSAC) of CCFA is the medical arm of the foundation and recommends to the Board of Trustees the direction of all research and education efforts. Physicians are appointed to the NSAC by its chairperson by virtue of their national prominence and expertise in the field of gastroenterology and inflammatory bowel disease (IBD). These physicians have a special responsibility to encourage support for CCFA and to further its goals within the medical community. They assist the lay leadership in the development of chapters and education programs. The NSAC is also responsible for all decisions concerning research awards.

Over the past 30 years, the NSAC has grown in size and stature under the leadership of nine chairmen, each of whom has left his individual legacy. Currently, the NSAC cabinet consists of ten active committees whose members represent both basic and clinical physicians and scientists from all across the United States.

CCFA's monetary commitment to research projects for 1998 is over $4 million. Current research projects cover a wide range of biomedical topics including epidemiology, immunology, genetics, infectious agents, microbiology, cancer, surgery, physiology, and clinical trials. Each year, the NSAC conducts peer reviews of 90 to 110 research grants and training award applications. Basic research grants are awarded on the basis of scientific merit and relevance to IBD. Projects are rated by the same scoring method used at the National Institutes of Health (NIH).

Grants are also awarded to variety of investigators including established researchers and newly independent researchers receiving first-time grants. Research training awards are given to promising new investigators at the beginning of their research careers to encourage them to enter the field of IBD research. CCFA's newest grant is the student research fellowship award where a stipend is provided for students to work in an accredited lab on a 10-week IBD research project.

Recently, exciting research areas have been identified and immediately supported, allowing the project to circumvent the lengthy standard grant review process. One such project was the mouse model of IBD developed at Jackson Laboratories in Maine, which has helped to revolutionize IBD research, along with the creation of a gene cell line and tissue bank.

All grant requests are submitted to the NSAC's grants council, which discusses and prioritizes all grant applications for their relevance to the "Challenges in IBD Research Agenda for the 1990s." This is a document that was created by more than 40 top researchers as a scientific blueprint for the direction and development of IBD research into the next century. Only upon the council's approval are the requests forwarded to CCFA's executive committee for funding.

The NSAC's clinical agenda committee has outlined the needs and defined the direction of clinical researchers, in much the same way as "Challenges in IBD Research Agenda for the 1990s" outlined the direction of basic research. Its first project is the formation of a clinical research network, which will link medical centers by computer across the country in order to study specific patient populations and/or drug effectiveness with greater ease. It will give clinicians and private practitioners an opportunity to produce quality clinical research ("at the bedside") from their own patient base. It will also allow practitioners to improve the standard of care for IBD patients while the basic scientists ("under the microscope") labor to find the cause and cure for their disease.

EDUCATION

"Education can turn the despair of having a chronic disease into hope and acceptance."

The Patient Education Committee of the NSAC is responsible for the development of educational materials on IBD for distribution to patients and their families, physicians, hospitals, schools, and libraries. Over the past few years, this committee has created several major books, three new brochures, video tapes, and a slide program for patient education in CCFA's chapters. It has also revised and updated the patient brochures. More than a million brochures are distributed, free of charge, each year. These dedicated physicians also work closely with the lay education leadership in creating how-to manuals for the chapters and programs of merit for the general public, as the "Coping Seminar" cookbook. A participatory educational program for patients suffering from CD and UC, their family members, and their friends, the coping seminar will assist them in learning ways to deal with the physical and emotional anguish of these disease and to improve their quality of life. Other valuable public education programs are planned at the chapter level involving local medical leaders and the chapter lay education leadership. Popular topics for chapter patient education meetings include the following:

Medical Overview for a Better Understanding of IBD
IBD Drug Therapy Including Effects and Side Effects of Medications
Extraintestinal Manifestations: IBD and the Effects on the Rest of
    the Body
Ostomies: Another Alternative
New Surgical Techniques
Surgical Alternatives and Procedures
When Is Surgery Necessary?
The Role of Nutrition in the Management of IBD
Dysplasia (Precancerous Cells) and Carcinoma in IBD

The Difference Between IBD and IBS (Irritable Bowel Syndrome)

What's New and What's Tried and True in Inflammatory Bowel Disease?

Etiology of IBD

When to Call the Doctor and How to Talk to Your Doctor

The Problem Colon and Dilemmas with Diarrhea

Choosing and Using Health Care Services

Chronic Pain in IBD and Its Effect on Family and Relationships

Coping with IBD

Diagnostic Tests and Procedures

Elemental Diets for IBD Patients

Enterostomal Therapy for Patients with Ostomies: Who, What, Where, and When?

Everything You Ever Wanted to Know About IBD but Were Afraid to Ask

Humor and Medicine: The Comic Spirit and Its Role in Health

IBD in Children: What Parents Can Do

Understanding Pediatric and Teenage IBD

Pediatric IBD: Social and Psychological Aspects

Role of the Family in IBD

Stress Management in IBD

Enteral and Parenteral Nutrition for IBD

Pediatric IBD: Social and Psychological Aspects

Role of the Family in IBD

Stress Management in IBD

Enteral and Parenteral Nutrition of IBD

Raising and Maintaining Self-Esteem in Patients with Chronic IBD

A Woman's Point of View: Sexuality and Pregnancy

Why CCFA Is Important to Patients with IBD

Your Rights as an IBD Patient

What's New in IBD Research

Update of Patients Rights at School and in the Workplace

Pediatric Surgery and New Developments in Treatment

Gender Differences in IBD

Discussing IBD with Others

Special Nutritional Needs with IBD Medications

General IBD Diet, Including Supplements and Total Parenteral
  Nutrition
Alternative Therapies for IBD

The Pediatric Affairs Committee of the NSAC develops programs
and materials to fill the needs of pediatric patients with IBD and the
medical professionals that care for them. Their recent publication,
Managing Your Child's Crohn's Disease or Ulcerative Colitis, is the
first complete pediatric resource for parents and families. Topic
include cause and diagnosis, review of drug and nondrug treatments,
surgery, diet and nutrition, school and social issues, hospitalization,
quality-of-life issues, and resources for the patient and family.
Another recent accomplishment for this committee is *Living with
IBD,* an educational booklet designed to help today's teenager better
understand and cope with CD and UC.

The Professional Education Committee of the NSAC concerns
itself with the education of the medical professional, bringing the
most current developments in the diagnosis and treatment of IBD,
which will, in turn, improve patient care throughout the country. This
committee is responsible for the creation of the successful medical
symposium available to CCFA chapters called the "Pathological and
Endoscopic Diagnosis in IBD Workshop Series," which has traveled
to many cities over the past few years. This road show has trained
thousands of pathologists, endoscopists, internists, general practitioners, and gastroenterologists throughout the country in working
together to diagnose CD and UC, with special attention given to dysplasia and cancer of the colon.

The most recent project from this committee is a symposium for
the nurse generalist entitled "Inflammatory Bowel Disease:
Update and Management." This course explores the definition and
differentiation of CD and UC, and covers the laboratory tests and
procedures used in the diagnosis of IBD and in its medical and
surgical treatment. An update on research in IBD is presented in
this program along with additional sessions on humor and medicine, management of ostomy patients, and the psychosocial issues
of living with IBD. The session ends with a panel discussion
composed of patients providing an opportunity for audience interaction.

COMMUNICATIONS

"Within 6 months in 1996, stories about IBD, CCFA, or individuals who have CD or UC reached more than 44 million people through the print media alone."

The editorial board of the NSAC started producing a small newsletter for its physician members called *IBD News*. Its popularity and circulation grew and it expanded to become *Progress in IBD*. But in 1995 this committee ceased its newsletter circulation to produce its own medical journal, *Inflammatory Bowel Diseases*. Available by subscription, the journal features high-quality, peer-reviewed articles from scientists all over the world who work at the cutting edge of IBD research. It has become enormously popular in the short time it has been in print and has been unanimously accepted by the medical community as the only journal devoted entirely to IBD.

Foundation Focus is the national magazine of the CCFA. Published 3 times yearly, this magazine contains articles of interest to our membership regarding research, medical therapy, and surgery. Regular features include messages from the president and the Chairman of the Board, Chapter News, Pharmacology Focus, and the popular "IBD File" section designed to educate the layperson on various topics relating to CD and UC.

In addition to *Foundation Focus,* the national membership receives newsletters from its local chapters. They serve as a means to keep the local membership informed of the success of recent and upcoming chapter events. These newsletters also feature articles by local physicians, chapter presidents, and the chapter executive director.

The yearly "Annual Report/Research Report" is a summary of CCFA's financial statements and current research awards. It was designed for prospective CCFA donors.

CCFA's Speakers Bureau comprises athletes, entertainers, and other celebrities who help raise funds and increase public awareness, as well as address a variety of chapter programs. Current members include actors Mary Ann Mobley, Mandy Patinkin, and John York; and athletes Rolf Benirskchke, Kevin Dineen, Peter Nielsen, and Trevor Wilson. These generous individuals help CCFA build a strong national image and raise needed dollars. The communications department serves as a liaison between the Speakers Bureau members and CCFA volunteers and staff. It develops national public service announcement campaigns and develops stories that are distributed to the national media (e.g., magazines and television talk shows).

CCFA's web site went live on the Internet in 1996. The web site address is <http://www.ccfa.org>. Features include the following: "Ask the Specialist," an online communication with CCFA physicians and other health care professionals; CCFA Library, a comprehensive database filled with media information and coping tips; "Progress in Research," with more than 155 articles on every major field of investigation; "News Updates," promoting major CCFA fund raising programs with information on research advances and new treatments; and "Write to CCFA," which enables members to send CCFA messages via computer. Virtually every single CCFA program, from local support groups and education programs to the tribute and memorial program, research grants, our brochures, and special events such as CCFA's "Pace Setter Walk," are included in this site. Within its first 2 years, individuals accessed CCFA's site over 6.5 million times, including hits from the United States and around the world.

SUPPORTIVE SERVICES

"Many individuals feel isolated with IBD until they attend a CCFA support group. Its goal is to create a warm, nonjudgmental atmosphere that invites members to share information and discuss their concerns."

CCFA provides national staff to answer patients' questions that come in by phone, via the 800-343-3637 hotline, or by mail. Some chapters also provide telephone support on a local level by trained volunteers who offer emotional support and information about IBD and CCFA. These volunteers follow the rules set up through CCFA's facilitator training program and are careful not to give medical advice.

Hospital visitation is another supportive service that many CCFA chapters offer. A qualified and trained patient volunteer serves as a role model to the hospital patient and as a positive representative of CCFA. Usually a patient is closely matched with a volunteer who has had a similar experience with IBD. This facilitates the understanding and communication between the hospitalized patient and the patient volunteer. The trained visitor follows the basic policies and procedures established by CCFA and visits the patient only with the permission of the patient's physician and the chapter's education chairperson or designee.

There are over 200 CCFA sponsored support groups throughout the United States. These groups are monitored by the local chapter education chairperson and are ultimately under the responsibility of the chapter executive director. CCFA's national education vice president and committee are currently working with the medical leadership in creating a uniform facilitator training and certification process for all CCFA sponsored support group volunteers.

Most of the 215 CCFA sponsored support groups meet monthly, in a moderately structured format, and a few meet on an 8-week basis with a more structured format addressing different topics each week. Both types of support groups include trained facilitators who act as gatekeepers to redirect discussion if it gets off track as well as to ensure that everyone has an opportunity to speak. CCFA's chapters offer educational medians where physicians and health care professionals address different topics. However, we find that patients express themselves more freely in support group sessions when professionals are not present. Most support groups do not charge a fee to attend the meetings; however, some groups do ask for a small contribution to offset the expense of each meeting, charging a lesser price if the participant is a CCFA member. However, no one should ever be turned away because of lack of funds. Participants should be allowed to make whatever contribution they can. While facilitators encourage group members to be open and honest, no one is permitted to dominate the session or to force someone to talk about a subject he or she would rather avoid.

Support groups can be very valuable. Because of the demographic mixture, group members have varied experiences, and they really help each other. Whatever problem someone is facing, there are nearly always others who have been there, serving as wonderful role models. People who have dealt with IBD for years can relate to children with IBD and can help parents understand what their kids go through. Understanding what friends and family also go through is an important part of support group. Though support groups have many benefits, we must recognize that some people are not comfortable in a support group. Some individuals get scared when they see others who are very sick. Others with acute illness may also feel out of place in a situation where some participants have only mild symptoms. And yet, there are others who prefer not to discuss intimate concerns in a group setting. However, most participants are enthusiastic and many make good friends on whom they can call day or night if need be.

In any group it is important to have guidelines. Guidelines enable participants to know what is expected and help them to feel comfortable in their group environment. One such guideline is that meetings should start and end on time, and this is carried at each meeting by facilitators. Another guideline is that discussions in CCFA support groups are confidential. The facilitators realize the importance of members showing mutual respect and of the participants feeling free to share personal experiences, information, and ideas. Medical advice is not to be given, nor should someone's management be critiqued. Following is a list of guidelines that the CCFA facilitator should mention at the beginning of each meeting to which all participants must adhere:

1. Patients can discuss the prescriptive medications they are taking but not the amount or dosage. They can simply refer to a high or low dose.
2. Physicians' names are not mentioned in the meeting. The CCFA chapter will be happy to provide a list of physician members to any patient.
3. Nonprescribed therapies of any kind should not be discussed or promoted in CCFA support groups.

INFORMATION ABOUT MONTHLY SUPPORT GROUPS

A comfortable size for a support group is around 12 people. For a monthly support group meeting, participants are free to attend every month or once a year. At one session, as many as 25 people may attend; at another, only 10. Most groups are mixed, incorporating men and women of all ages, newly diagnosed and long-time patients, people with mild disease and those with acute symptoms. Many also include a significant other or parents. Chapters may adapt their programs to meet the special needs of their members. Some chapters have support groups for people who have had ostomy surgery, teens, parents, and gay men.

Many groups do not establish topics for discussion in advance. The group sits around a conference table or in a circle, and the facilitator usually introduces himself or herself, giving a brief personal history of the disease and ending with why he or she is involved with the CCFA support group. The leader then goes around the room, asking participants how they have been doing in their own life. Most people feel comfortable about expressing their concerns about their disease, yet some are naturally shy and prefer to limit their discussion, preferring to listen. The trained leader will attempt to draw out responses and encourage participation without pressuring anyone to reply. A trained leader is also aware that this may be the first time some patients have had the opportunity to openly discuss their illness. Leaders will encourage people to talk while at the same time discouraging graphic accounts that tend to frighten newly diagnosed patients. They will also stop people from monopolizing the meeting. Group participation should be a positive experience for all involved.

There are unique concerns expressed by new facilitators in newly formed CCFA support groups. After the group is underway and members are beginning to get to know each other, new group leaders may worry that there might not be enough to talk about in group sessions or that there may be long, uncomfortable silences. Although experience with IBD support groups has shown that there is more than enough to talk about, some new leaders may feel more comfortable with a list of possible topics to introduce. The following topics have been used by support groups in some CCFA chapters. The questions that follow can be used to help stimulate discussion.

Reaction of Friends and Family

Who is your support system? How did your support system react when you were first diagnosed? Were you given erroneous advice from friends and well-wishers about the nature of your illness? (Many group members may have been told their disease was due to stress or poor eating habits, etc.) Is it easy to ask for help when you need it? How does your support system react to long bouts of flare-ups? Do sick youngsters get more attention from their parents? How does that create problems in the family?

Coping with a Chronic Illness

Share strategies of coping. For example, do you check ahead to find out where the bathrooms are located? Do you order a meal for your dietary needs in advance of a banquet function or business meeting? Is it a good idea to carry a change of clothes at all times? Should you talk to teachers on behalf of a child to ensure that child's immediate access to toilet facilities, etc.? What do you do if you have an accident?

Feelings About Medical Treatment

How do you feel about surgery, tests, and having to take medicines such as prednisone? What are the effects of prednisone on your mood, your appearance, the way you feel about yourself? How do you feel about trying new medications?

Feelings About Sex

Do you have fears about something happening during sexual intercourse? Do you have fears of being unattractive or about having children? Do you avoid intimacy because of these feelings or because of the IBD pain? How can an unmarried person be open with a prospective mate without scaring him or her off? How do you explain the side effects of medication to a friend or mate?

Impact of IBD on Lifestyle

Can you work, go to school, take vacation, go out with friends? Have you missed work days or classes? How have the employers or teachers reacted to your illness? If you are single, can you have a normal social life? Are there certain precautions you can take if you know you will be traveling for a long time without having access to a bathroom? Is your life sometimes dependent on where the bathroom is? Can you be open about that need, or must it be a secret?

Reaction to Having Chronic Illness

What does it feel like to find out, perhaps midway through life, that you have a chronic illness? How did you find out, and what were your early symptoms? Did you get the right diagnosis the first time? How does the mood-altering effect of medications affect you, your daily life, and your relationships?

Other Topics

Physical Activity and IBD
Using the Illness to Cop Out
Traveling with IBD
Role of the Family in IBD
Why CCFA Is Important
Complications of IBD (Extraintestinal Manifestations)
Fighting Depression
Dealing with Your Physician
Coping with Illness (at home/work/school, and with family/friends/
  co-workers/schoolmates)
Family/Friends Support (how they do or do not help you deal with
  IBD)
Feelings about Surgery and Tests
Five Phases of Chronic Illness (denial, anger, hope, depression,
  acceptance)
Diet

Note: Because nutritional needs vary, questions about vitamin therapy, nutritional deficiencies, and nutritional supplements should be referred to the patient's gastroenterologist.

SUGGESTED 8-WEEK PROGRAM FOR CCFA SUPPORT GROUPS

Some chapters prefer to offer support groups on an 8-week session. Usually these sessions take place each year in the fall and in the spring. Ideally, groups meet once a week for 8 weeks and the meetings last 2 hours. These groups may be limited to 12 members, plus 2 leaders. Usually these groups charge a small fee for the 8-week session (e.g., $15 per participant). Any of the topics suggested for monthly support group meetings can be discussed during the 8-week program. The suggestion for the 8-week program can be followed, or it can be redesigned to meet the needs of any support group.

Week 1: Introductions

Moderators introduce themselves and give short background of CCFA and the support group program. The ground rules are discussed. Then each patient in turn is asked to give a short introduction, including name, occupation, marital status (if they wish), interests, etc. On the second time around the circle the patient identifies his or her illness, its onset, severity, and current status. The moderator explains that he or she is a nonprofessional. The purpose of the group is a rap session, informally led, in which all members are asked to participate but no professional advice is given. Experiences will be shared to find just how much the group has in common. Such topics as early symptoms, what it feels like to have a chronic illness, what "chronic" means, whether your disease was diagnosed correctly the first time, and whether you were ill prior to the first severe attack might be covered. At this first session patients start to get to know each other.

Week 2: Support Systems/Reaction of Friends and Family

Reactions to the first week are discussed. Was the group excited? Disappointed? (Many come hoping to get a lot of medical information and may be disappointed that it is not forthcoming.) Did they share their experience with anyone? Who is your support system? Is it a parent, spouse, sibling, or friend? What were the reactions of friends and family? How did you get to the doctor who diagnosed your illness? Were you given erroneous advice about the nature of your illness by friends and well-wishers? (At least half of past group members have been told that their disease was emotionally based, due to stress or poor eating habits, etc.) Have you had experiences in trying to share your problem with another who did not understand or wish to hear it? How does that feel?

Week 3: Impact of IBD on Lifestyle

Any unfinished business from the prior week is always discussed first. How has your illness affected your lifestyle? This topic addresses the same questions as the monthly support group.

Week 4: Sharing Feelings About the Doctor

Feeling are shared about the doctor–patient relationship, without mentioning any physician by name or location, or hospital affiliation, that includes both positive and negative relationships. Is your doctor available to you? Does he or she answer all of your questions? Do you feel he or she may be holding back? Has your doctor informed you about the possible side effects of your medication? Does your doctor spend time with you on the phone? Was this the first doctor you have seen, and how did you get to him or her? Is he or she available in the event of an emergency? What kind of tests did you need? How often do you see your doctor? What about x-rays and sigmoidoscopy, colonoscopy? How do you get good medical care if you can't afford a private physician? If you belong to a group health plan, can you get proper treatment?

Weeks 5–8: Sharing Feelings About the Surgery, etc.

Feelings about surgery, medical treatment, diagnostic tests, and the increased possibility of cancer are discussed. Feelings about dependency and independence, sex, the fear of being unattractive, and the possibility of children inheriting the illness are discussed. Finally, coping techniques, both practical and emotional, are covered.

Having CD or UC can be confusing, unsettling, and sometimes overwhelming. The loss of control over one's self can be very humbling. With the exchange of information, group support can sometimes bring an understanding of one's own feelings, with insight into one's own behavior and that of others. In knowing that you are not alone, it is sometimes easier to accept limitations. In this way you can learn to control your disease somewhat rather than have the disease control you.

The development and current structure of CCFA's supportive services can be credited to many chapter volunteers and staff throughout the United States, with special recognition of the efforts of the Greater New York Chapter, the Georgia Chapter, the Houston/Gulf Coast Chapter, and the Michigan Chapter.

HOW TO TALK TO YOUR DOCTOR

"Exercising your right to participate in decisions about your treatment and becoming more assertive in communications with your physician can help you achieve a level of independence that most patients want."

The patient–physician relationship is just as important to the well-being of persons with IBD as their home environment and the medications they take. A patient's interaction with a physician is an integral component of coping with the disease. There are a few simple guidelines to remember that will help you talk with your doctor:

1. Remember that your conversations with your physician are confidential, so feel safe to be open about your symptoms of IBD and your concerns. Most doctors are compassionate.
2. Always be honest with your doctor, so that the trust is mutual. Following instructions that you both agree to also builds trust (e.g., taking your medicine).
3. Before visiting your doctor, write down your questions so that you do not forget to ask what is on your mind.
4. Take an active role in being a partner in your treatment of IBD instead of simply following instructions. If you have concerns about what your physician says, let him or her know it right away, as there may be an alternative to which you can both agree.
5. Become educated about your illness. It is your responsibility to take advantage of the educational materials and programs offered by the CCFA and it will help in understanding and reinforcing your physician's words.

CONCLUSION

"As people with CD or UC, we can live life to its fullest."

Some people diagnosed with IBD cope very well. Yet others struggle in their daily lives, just tolerating the humbling symptoms of active bowel disease. They may take medications that bring undesirable side effects. The IBD may interrupt school, work, and social or recreational activities. Relationships with well-meaning friends and family may become strained. Life with CD or UC can be overwhelming. We may experience any of the following emotions:

Despair	Pain
Lack of energy	Humbleness
Fearfulness	Stress
Depression	Anger
Isolation	Denial
Loneliness	Frustration
Lack of control	

Acting on our behalf, CCFA is busy raising funds and supporting research to find the cause and the cure of IBD, and working to dispel the ignorance of the public about CD and UC. During periods of disease activity, you can:

1. Lean on the CCFA for support in helping you cope with IBD.
2. Become informed about your disease through CCFA's educational materials and local programs.
3. Act responsibly with your disease and medications.
4. Work with your physician as a partner in fighting your illness.
5. Look to your inner self for strength and have hope for a remission.

When the CD or the UC responds to drug therapy we begin to feel better. When overcoming the adversity of IBD we may experience joy about being in remission, and happiness to function in a normal way.

As patients, we can reach out by partnering with CCFA to break the mold. We may even find happiness by helping others to cope with IBD. And last, we will accept the things we cannot change, e.g., the disease, surgery, life with medication, while looking ahead to the bright future!

APPENDIX

Patient Resources and Materials Available

CCFA's toll-free hotline: 800-343-3637
CCFA's national headquarters:

Crohn's and Colitis Foundation of America, Inc.
386 Park Avenue South, 17th Floor
New York, NY 10016-8804
(212) 685-3440 phone
(212) 779-4098 fax
CCFA's web site: http://www.ccfa.org

Brochures Available Free of Charge

Questions and Answers about Crohn's Disease
Questions and Answers about Ulcerative Colitis
*Preguntas y Reputation Acerca de la Enfermedad Crohn and
    Colitis ulcerativa*
Questions and Answers about Diet and Nutrition
Questions and Answers about Pregnancy
Questions and Answers about Complications
Crohn's Disease, Ulcerative Colitis, and Your Child
*A Guide for Children and Teenagers to Crohn's Disease and
    Ulcerative Colitis*
Questions and Answers about Emotional Factors
A Teacher's Guide to Crohn's Disease and Ulcerative Colitis
Questions and Answers about Surgery
Medications for Inflammatory Bowel Disease

Books Available
(check local chapters or national headquarters for prices)

The New People...Not Patients: A Source Book for Living with IBD
*Treating IBD: A Patient's Guide to the Medical and Surgical
    Management*
Managing Your Child's Crohn's Disease and Ulcerative Colitis
*Inflammatory Bowel Disease: A Guide for Patients and Their
    Families*

Membership

Includes national magazine *Foundation Focus* (3 issues per year)
    and local chapter newsletter
Minimum $25 per year for individual membership (contact CCFA)

GLOSSARY OF MEDICAL TERMS

abscess: a pocket or collection of pus. In IBD these typically form in the abdominal cavity or rectal area.

ankylosis: fusion of the bones of the spinal column.

anticholinergic: a class of drugs that can relax the smooth muscle of the intestine.

autoimmunity: an inflammatory reaction to one's own tissues.

clinical: involving the direct observation and treatment of patients.

contraindication: any circumstance making a form of medical or surgical treatment unadvisable.

dermatitis: irritation or inflammation of the skin.

edema: accumulation of excessive amounts of fluid in the tissues that may result in swelling.

electrolytes: acids, bases, and salts essential for maintaining life.

endoscopy: direct examination of the interior of the digestive tract using a fiberoptic endoscope, such as a sigmoidoscope, colonoscope, or gastroscope.

epidemiology: the study of the frequency and distribution of diseases in the population.

exacerbation: an increase in symptoms or reactivation of disease; a relapse.

fissure: a crack or crevice in the skin surrounding the anus.

fistula: an abnormal channel connecting two structures, e.g., adjacent loops of intestine or the intestine and another structure such as the bladder, vagina, or skin.

fluoroscopy: a type of x-ray examination in which the shadows of organs being examined are made visible on a screen.

folic acid: one of the vitamins responsible for the formation of red blood cells.

fulminant: with extreme rapidity.

gut: general term for intestine or bowel.

idiopathic: of unknown cause.

immunology: study of the body's immune response to disease.

immunomodulatory agents or immunosuppressive agents: drugs that suppress the body's immune response to disease or environmental agents.

inflammation: a process characterized by pain, redness, heat, and swelling.

inflammatory mediators: powerful chemicals released by the body as part of the inflammatory response.

intractable: unrelieved by medical treatment.

lactose intolerance: a condition caused by a decrease or absence of the enzyme lactase, which aids in digestion of milk sugar.

leukotrienes: powerful chemical mediators released during the inflammatory process that promote the movement of white blood cells to the site of inflammation.

lumen: the interior of a hollow organ, such as the intestine.

mucus: a whitish substance normally produced by the intestine and that may be found in increased amounts in the stool when the intestine is diseased.

osteonecrosis: death of bone tissue. This may result from use of long-term high-dose steroids.

oxalate stones: kidney stones formed from calcium oxalate and found in IBD patients with fat malabsorption resulting from ileal disease or resection.

oxygen radicals: toxic products of oxygen metabolism that may cause tissue damage in IBD.

paresthesias: abnormal sensations in the feet and lower legs, often felt as pins and needles.

pathogen: a microorganism (bacterium or virus) capable of causing disease.

pathogenesis: the origin and development of disease.

perineal: involving the anal and genital areas and their surrounding tissues.

prolapse: the falling or protrusion of an organ, such as the rectum or stoma.

prostaglandin: another inflammatory mediator that may cause the intestine to lose fluid and electrolytes, resulting in diarrhea.

protein-losing enteropathy: loss of circulating proteins and other nutrients through the inflamed bowel wall.

remission: a reduction of symptoms and a return to good health.

sepsis: infection of the bloodstream with microorganisms.

spondylitis: arthritis of the spine.

thrombophlebitis: inflammation and clotting of veins.

GLOSSARY OF SURGICAL TERMS

adhesions: scar tissue. In IBD these often connect two adjacent loops of intestine or a section of intestine to the abdominal wall, and can be associated with bowel obstruction.

anastomosis: a surgical connection.

catheter: a thin tube placed in a body cavity, organ, or vessel for the purpose of administering or draining fluids.

colostomy: a surgically created opening of the colon to the abdominal wall, allowing the diversion of fecal waste.

colectomy: a surgical removal of all or part of the colon.

distal: closer to the anus; downstream.

drains: catheters placed around areas where bowel has been removed to collect and drain fluids and prevent wound infection.

excision: surgical removal.

hemorrhage: abnormally heavy bleeding.

ileostomy: a surgically created opening of the ileum to the abdominal wall, allowing the diversion of fecal waste.

nasogastric tube: a flexible tube passed through the nose or mouth into the stomach. This tube is necessary to aspirate fluids and air that collect in the stomach when the bowel is obstructed or after gastrointestinal surgery.

obstruction: a blockage of the small or large intestine preventing the normal passage of intestinal contents.

percutaneous: through the skin.

perforation: formation of a hole in the bowel wall, allowing intestinal contents to enter the peritoneal cavity.

peristalsis: wave-like muscular movements that propel food through the digestive tract.

peristomal: the area immediately surrounding the stoma.

peritoneum: the membrane that encloses the abdominal organs, forming the peritoneal or abdominal cavity.

peritonitis: inflammation or infection of the peritoneum, usually resulting from an intestinal perforation.

proctectomy: surgical removal of the rectum. This would require the formation of either an internal pouch or an ileostomy.

proctocolectomy: removal of the entire colon and rectum.

proximal: closer to the mouth; upstream.

resection: surgical removal of a diseased portion of intestine.

reservoir: a surgically created pouch made from the distal ileum to collect intestinal waste.

sphincter: a ring of muscle tissue keeping certain sections of the digestive tract (such as the anus) closed.

stenosis: a narrowing.

stoma: a surgically created opening of the bowel onto the skin, the result of ostomy surgery.

stricture: a narrowed area of intestine caused by active inflammation or scar tissue.

subtotal colectomy: removal of part or most of the colon, leaving a part (usually the rectum) intact.

sutures: materials used in surgery to rejoin cut tissues and close wounds.

Subject Index

Page numbers followed by *f* refer to figures; page numbers followed by *t* refer to tables.

A

Abdominal pain
 bowel obstruction causing, 151
 CD causing, 41, 150
 children with, 81
 UC causing, 32
Acupuncture as therapy,
  185–186
Adolescents. *See* Children and
  adolescents
Adrenocorticotropic hormone
  (ACTH) treating CD, 48
African-Americans with IBD, 24
Alcohol
 folic acid absorption inhibited
  by, 18
 liver metabolizing, 13
 pancreatitis caused by, 12
Alternative medicine. *See also*
  Integrated medicine
 consumer use of, 176
 doctors' response to, 176
 FDA policy toward, 186
 gastroenterologist, choice
  of, 176
 herbal remedies. *See*
  Herbal remedies
 insurance coverage for,
  178–179
 medical training for, 179–182
 overview of, 175–178
 physical therapies, 184–190.
  See also specific types,
  e.g. Yoga as therapy

Amebiasis, IBD mistaken
  for, 81
Aminosalicylates
 azo-linked agents, 127
 doses of, 128*t*
 enemas of, 126
 indications for, 128*t*
 oral forms of, 126
 side effects of, 127
 slow-release agents, 126
 topical forms of, 125–126
 UC treated by, 34
Anal skin
 sensitivity of, 166
 tabs, 42, 166, 173
Anastomosis. *See also*
  J-pouch
 ileorectal, 158*f*
 small bowel, 153
 small intestine, 167
Anemia
 folic acid deficiency
  causing, 18
 nutritional loss causing, 101
 UC causing, 37
Antibiotics. *See also*
  specific types
 breastfeeding affected by, 73
 CD treated by, 40, 51
 generally, 134–136
 pregnancy affected by, 73
Anticholinergic agents, 138
Antidepressants, 138
Antituberculous agents, 136